FACT OR MYTH?

- Women on the Pill are at greater risk of incurring a yeast infection.
- Taking antibiotics increases your chances of getting a yeast infection.
- You can fight infection by eating "good" bacteria.
- Using tampons instead of sanitary napkins can help prevent yeast infections.
- Diaper rash can be a sign of yeast infection in infants.
- Garlic helps cure a yeast infection.

All these statements are true. Find out more about this troublesome health problem and what you can do to help yourself in:

A Woman's Guide to Yeast Infections

NAOMI BAUMSLAG, M.D., M.P.H., is the founder and president of the Women's International Public Health Network, a nonprofit organization devoted to addressing women's issues in public health and improving the health of women worldwide. She is a clinical professor of pediatrics and community medicine and family health at Georgetown University Medical School. She also serves as an international health consultant.

DIA L. MICHELS is a professional writer and consultant. She has done numerous articles and interviews on medical topics.

ABOUT THE AUTHORS

Naomi Baumslag is cofounder and president of the Women's International Public Health Network (WIPHN). She is also a clinical professor at Georgetown University School of Medicine. She has published numerous scientific articles and authored five books. Her books include *Mother and Child Health: Delivering the Services* (Oxford University) and *Breastfeeding: The Passport to Life* (UNICEF). Dr. Baumslag earned her M.D. at the University of Witwatersrand in South Africa and holds a Masters in Public Health from Johns Hopkins University School of Hygiene and Public Health. She has testified before Congress and received awards for her contributions in the areas of women and child health. She has three children and lives with her husband in Bethesda, Maryland.

Dia L. Michels is a researcher and writer specializing in health topics relating to women. In addition to working with Dr. Baumslag on this book, they are collaborating on a book examining the history, culture, and politics of breast-feeding. Ms. Michels is also developing children's educational books and materials. She teaches and lectures, and has written and produced a weekly radio show on women's issues. A graduate of Brandeis University, she also studied in Scotland and France. She lives with her husband and daughter in Washington, D.C.

A WOMAN'S GUIDE TO YEAST INFECTIONS

Naomi Baumslag, M.D., and Dia L. Michels

POCKET BOOKS

New York   London   Toronto   Sydney   Tokyo   Singapore

An important part of informed self-care is knowing when to seek out your community's health-care resources. Readers should consult a physician or professional health-care provider on a regular basis; such consultation should be immediately sought if you have or suspect you have any condition which may require professional diagnosis or medical attention.

This book is not meant to be a substitute for regular visits to your doctor or the treatment given by your doctor. It was written as a general informational guide and reference source. No medical or legal responsibility is assumed by the authors.

An *Original* Publication of POCKET BOOKS

POCKET BOOKS, a division of Simon & Schuster Inc.
1230 Avenue of the Americas, New York, NY 10020

ISBN: 0-671-74699-5

First Pocket Books printing June 1992

10 9 8 7 6 5 4 3 2 1

POCKET and colophon are registered trademarks of
Simon & Schuster Inc.

Cover design by Gina Bonanno
Illustrations by Jeffrey L. Ward

Printed in the U.S.A.

To Tony,
who gave me a writer's chair—
and encouraged me to sit in it.
—DLM

Acknowledgments

Many people helped us make this book a reality. We'd like to thank our agent, Bill Adler, Jr., and our editor at Pocket Books, Claire Zion, for helping us bring the book to the public.

Particular thanks go to Ralph Yodaiken, M.D., Doyle Niemann, Jordan Michels, D.C., Patrick Meehan, M.D., and Laura Kane. We'd also like to thank Rene Smit, C.N.M., Jean Godwin, Leo Sreebny, D.D.S., M.S., Ph.D., Michael Sanders, Kevin Remmers, Sudhanvshu Pethe, Michael Connelly, Cindy Scharf, Philip Zimmerman, Ph.D., Lawrence R. Siegel, R.P.H., Mark Ponds, R.P.H., Michele and Wally Dicks, and Blanca Keogan.

And special thanks go to all the women who took time to share their experiences and concerns with us.

CONTENTS

PREFACE   xiii

INTRODUCTION   1

Why Women? / 5
The Terminology / 7
History of Yeast Infections / 8
The Incidence of Yeast Infections Is Rising
   Sharply / 11
A Vicious Cycle / 12
Where Do We Go from Here? / 15
New Hope—An Effective Treatment
   Program / 16

PART ONE
UNDERSTANDING YEAST

1 ALL ABOUT FUNGI: 21
A KINGDOM ALL THEIR OWN

Candida Albicans / 31
Fungal Infections in Perspective / 33

2 YEAST TRIGGERS   35

Antibiotic Therapy / 40
Another Source of Antibiotics / 42

Oral Contraceptives / 44
Poor Menstrual Management / 47
Pregnancy, Childbirth, and Breast-feeding / 49
Sexual Transmission / 52
*Sexual Transmissibility: Oral, Anal, and Lesbian
   Sex* / 58
General Abrasions/Irritations / 60
Immunosuppressant Therapy / 62
*Other Weaknesses in the Immune System: Illness,
   Poor Nutrition, Stress* / 64
Infancy / 66

3 A PRIMER ON VAGINITIS   70

The Myths of Yeast Infections:
1. *Use of the Pill is not related to your chronic
   yeast infections* / 71
2. *You can't catch it from, or give it to, a sexual
   partner* / 73
3. *If you just wait, your menstrual cycle will
   "cleanse out" the infection* / 75
4. *Women with any type of vaginal problem
   should never wear tampons* / 77
5. *Yeast infections will go away by themselves if
   just ignored* / 78
6. *Yeast infections are simply a normal part of
   being female* / 79
7. *All women with recurring vaginitis should be
   tested for diabetes* / 80
8. *Intermittent prophylactic therapy is the best
   treatment approach* / 81
When Is Yeast Responsible for the Infection / 82
Vaginitis / 87
Guidelines for Avoiding Vaginitis / 103
*Yeast Infections as Indicators of Other
   Problems* / 104

4 WHEN SHOULD YOU GO TO A DOCTOR?
109

THE PHYSICAL AND EMOTIONAL ASPECTS OF YEAST INFECTIONS

What to Expect / 112
The Traditional Medical Approach / 117
The Emotional Chaos / 123

PART TWO
TREATING YEAST

5 GETTING FREE
133

Point 1: Strengthen Your Overall Health / 135
Point 2: Build Up Your Yeast-Controlling Bacteria / 137
Point 3: Reduce the Yeast Population in the Vagina / 143
Point 4: Reduce the Yeast Population of the Gastrointestinal Tract / 144
Treating Yourself / 149
  Home Remedies / 151
  Antifungal Drug Treatments / 172
  Nondrug Antifungal Agents / 183
  Treatment and Prevention for the Partner / 191
  Treatment for Special Cases / 196
  Treatments of the Future / 208

6 STAYING FREE
211

General Prevention Tips / 213
Specific Prevention Tips / 225
The Yeast-Free Diet / 234
Guide to Taking Antibiotics / 237

APPENDICES   241

A. Glossary of Medical Terms / 241
B. List of Broad-Spectrum and Narrow-Spectrum
   Antibiotics / 244
C. Suggested Reading / 247
D. The FDA Hearings: June 1990 / 249

REFERENCES AND NOTES   255

INDEX   263

PREFACE

For centuries, women were considered the weaker sex, their health ignored, their medical problems blamed on their gender, temperament, or hormones. Women were expected to suffer their "womanly ills" in silence. In large part, this has contributed to the lack of interest and research in women's health, exemplified by the paucity of information on the pathogenesis of yeast infections and the effectiveness of many drug and home remedies. This is largely due to the lack of randomized, controlled clinical trials.

Vaginal yeast infections are out of the closet. In the U.S. alone, over 22 million women each year are affected. Three out of every four women will have a yeast infection in their lifetime, and the rate of recurrence is high.

Prescription vaginal yeast infection drugs are big business: 1990 sales totalled $220 million, exclusive of the millions more spent on nonprescription treatments. Sales of vaginal over-the-counter (OTC) yeast medications are expected to top $400 million by 1995. With so much money at stake, it's no wonder that women and doctors are wooed by a myriad of advertisements featuring products promising cure.

We wrote this book to help women understand, prevent, and take steps to treat their yeast infections.

Each woman's circumstances are different, and, unfortunately, we have no magic bullet. The treatments discussed here include not only modern medical approaches, but also homeopathic and home remedies, as well as nutritional guidelines.

This book is not intended to replace your doctor; it is intended to provide you with the knowledge and tools to make informed health-care decisions.

—N. BAUMSLAG and D. MICHELS
May 1991

INTRODUCTION

•

If I had a nickel for every yeast infection I've had,
I'd be a rich woman right now.

—29-year-old woman in Syracuse

*V*aginal yeast infections are messy and nasty and painful. No one likes to talk about them, yet they plague
millions of women—not just once, but over and over
again.

What is a yeast infection? It is a common inflammation of the vagina caused by an overgrowth of the
organism Candida albicans, a type of yeast normally
present in a healthy vagina. Typical symptoms include
vaginal itching; a white discharge, resembling cottage
cheese and sometimes with a yeasty smell like that of
baking bread; a reddened, swollen vaginal area; and a
burning sensation, especially when urinating or having
intercourse.

Candida albicans, candidal vulvovaginitis, monilial
vaginitis, chronic candidiasis—call it what you will,
but no matter the label, these vaginal yeast infections
strike record numbers of women every day of the year.
While these diseases occur predominantly during a
woman's reproductive years, women between the ages
of 15 and 45 are not the only victims. Infants may pick
up yeast passing through the birth canal, and adolescent girls can get it, especially after antibiotic treatment. Heterosexual and lesbian women may be infected by their lovers, since the disease can be sexually
transmitted. Outbreaks among nuns in convents have

been reported, too, and postmenopausal women may become susceptible from the hormonal imbalance.

Who knows better the pain and misery that yeast infections cause in women across the land than the doctors who treat these women daily.

> During the last twenty years the frequency has steadily increased and Candida albicans is now the most frequently known cause of vulvovaginitis. . . . A primary cure rate of about 90 percent has been recorded for a wide range of preparations. However, within a few months, relapse/reinfection frequencies of up to 30 percent have been reported.
>
> —Merete Leegaard,
> *Acta Obstetrical Gynecology of Scandinavia*

> . . . it has been estimated that up to 75 percent of women will have at least one episode of candidal vaginitis during their reproductive years and half of them will have multiple episodes . . .
>
> —Jack Sobel,
> *New England Journal of Medicine*

> 15–20 percent of all women have chronic recurrent vulvovaginal candidiasis with attacks every month.
>
> —Trowbridge/Walker,
> *The Yeast Syndrome*

Fully one-third of all visits to gynecologists are prompted by a vaginal discharge, and a yeast infection is one of the most frequent diagnoses. Doctors then prescribe creams, suppositories, and ointments to eradicate the condition. Though usually successful in removing the symptoms, these treatments often don't eliminate the problem. Studies in the U.S., England,

Western Europe, and Scandinavia report recurrence rates ranging from 25 to 75 percent. A review of the past 20 years of medical research on yeast infections from around the globe unveils the same three words over and over: *Recurrence is common*.

For many women, the cycle of yeast infections takes on a life of its own: pain, itching, and discomfort; a trip to the gynecologist; creams, suppositories, and ointments; and then more infection and more treatment, on and on. With each new outbreak, the underlying condition becomes more entrenched, the financial outlay increases, the emotional frustration rises, and the condition becomes ever harder to eradicate.

From a slightly different angle, yeast infections represent more than just a frequent complaint, they are an expensive one as well. Each visit to the doctor generates an office fee, an exam fee, and fees for laboratory tests, not to mention what you might spend for a follow-up visit. The medications can cost up to $30 per course; and often, two to three courses are prescribed. When the price tag for one infection can easily be hundreds of dollars, it's easy to see how the cost for recurrent infections can pass the thousand-dollar mark in no time at all, a boon to both the medical establishment and the pharmaceutical companies. That's a lot of consumer dollars for what is often referred to as a "minor feminine irritation!"

Understandably, women get very frustrated with the doctors' inability to eradicate the condition. After several trips to the gynecologist, women often end up scanning the shelves of health food and book stores in search of alternative therapies. The market has responded accordingly with a plethora of products and publications, some effective, some not, aimed at the female self-care audience. The most common result, however, is more confusion and still lighter pocketbooks.

These infections drain the emotions as well as the purse. When women complain, doctors all too frequently respond with dismissive remarks: "You must be using it wrong"; "These drugs work for everyone else"; or "Certain people have tendencies to certain problems, and this is simply one you'll have to learn to live with." These same doctors, however, rarely, if ever, mention prevention. The most common advice they give is to use the medications every time there is the first sign of an infection and continue until well after it's gone; advice that translates into staying on the medications two to three weeks each month. Physicians may trivialize recurrence, brush aside the inconvenience of constant treatment, ignore the cost of medication, and minimize the associated physical and emotional pain. As a result, millions of women are spending millions of dollars and untold hours each year vigorously treating yeast infections with only limited success.

Where can a woman turn for advice on coping with recurrent yeast infections? The information women need to free themselves from this painful and emotionally debilitating cycle of infection is well hidden. The available self-help general health books deal with the subject only briefly or, when specifically taking intestinal yeast overgrowth as their subject promote a speculative theory, recommend obscure therapies, and are almost exclusively written by men. Altogether, these books offer little to the woman struggling with recurrent yeast vaginitis. While there is a significant amount of medical literature on alleviating chronic vaginal yeast infections, they are not widely available or easily accessible to most of us.

We wrote this book for all the women eager to play a larger, more educated role in their own health care. It is designed for women who have an occasional infection as well as for those who, feeling frustrated and alone, have been searching for answers in vain. In it, we provide the background information you need to understand what questions to ask, and then how to answer those questions. This book provides a four-step approach to vaginal yeast infections. It will allow you to get a handle on this annoying condition whether you have sporadic infections or recurrent episodes.

Why Women?

Why is it that women hold such a monopoly on yeast infections? Yeast organisms cause a wide variety of diseases in a number of diverse environments. The most commonly affected sites on the human body are the mouth, the vagina, the anal canal, and the nails. It's not that men don't get yeast infections; they are susceptible to oral thrush and jock itch, as well as far more serious systemic yeast conditions. But vaginal yeast infections are exceptionally common and women do obviously have exclusivity on these.

Yeast organisms need a place to live, and from their point of view, women of childbearing age are superior hostesses. A woman's body offers an ideal nesting ground for yeast organisms satisfying, as it does, three crucial criteria for their growth. First, the anatomy of the vagina provides yeast with a perfect breeding arena. It is warm (yeast loves temperatures found in tropical climates), and it is moist (yeast cannot survive without a high degree of relative humidity). Normally, the vagina is a relatively tranquil area of the body, well protected against major disturbances. Yet it is also close enough to the anus, a reservoir of yeast colonies, so that contamination of the vagina with fresh spores is possible.

Second, the normal female hormones actually create a chemical environment conducive to yeast growth. A positive relationship between hormones and

Candida vulvovaginitis has long been recognized. The high incidence of infection occurring during pregnancy, in women using oral contraceptives, and in the premenstrual period, along with its relative rarity before puberty and after menopause (unless estrogen-replacement hormones are taken) provides a clear picture of a hormone/Candida link.

Finally, the vagina can be a site of some pretty exciting events. Changes in the local environment resulting from sexual stimulation, the arrival of semen, and the regular presence of nutritious menstrual blood all encourage yeast growth. Between the anatomy, the hormones, and the regular changes in the local environment, the vaginal region gives a veritable red-carpet welcome to yeasts. No area of a man's body can compare.

Once the field of yeast sufferers has been narrowed down to the female half of the population, further narrowing proves elusive. It is difficult to accurately predict who the likely sufferers will be. Why some women develop recurring episodes while others are never affected remains obscure. Breaking women into categories by income, educational background, occupation, number of sexual partners, race, marital status, or number of children unveils few similarities. Many women struggling with yeast infections have no known predisposing factors and no easy culprit can be isolated as having "caused" the infection.

Poor women find themselves with their fair share of yeast infections, potentially due to a compromised nutritional state (malnutrition is a predisposing factor). On the other hand, wealthy women are not spared, most likely due to the fact that wealthy women visit doctors more, and therefore receive a disproportionate amount of prescriptions for such drugs as antibiotics and immunosuppressants (known triggers for yeast infections). Sexually active women get their fair share of yeast infections, but then the higher the degree of sexual activity, the greater the incidence of genital infections of all kinds. Alternatively, some of the more persistent cases of candidal vaginitis have been found in virgins and there is even evidence of yeast infections among nuns in convents. Yeast infections are seen most commonly in women of childbearing age, but this group does not hold exclusivity. In fact, the first written report of candida vaginitis was in a seventy-seven-year-old woman; and intravaginal antifungal prescriptions for four-year-olds have been required. Study after study has attempted to identify the vulnerable groups, but indeed, just about the only requirement for a vaginal yeast infection seems to be being female.

The Terminology

Before we proceed any further, it's worth spending a little time to understand the terminology. Our concern is with vaginal yeast infections, specifically those infections caused by the organism known as *Candida albicans*. The medical condition caused by this organism is often referred to with a term incorporating the infecting agent's name—*candidiasis, candidasis, candidiosis,* or *candidosis* (the different suffixes all mean a "condition" or "state of"). Practitioners tried to distinguish between the use of the *asis* terms versus the *osis* terms, with one referring to the presence of yeast and the other referring to the presence of infection caused by yeast. This distinction never took hold; all the terms are now used interchangeably. Generally speaking, candidiasis is more commonly used by Americans; Canadians, British, French, and Italians tend to prefer candidosis.

Other terms used commonly include *thrush, mycosis, monilia, moniliasis,* and *vaginitis.* Infections of the mucous membranes, typically in the vagina or mouth, caused by yeasts are regularly referred to as thrush (often clarified by a descriptor, such as vaginal thrush or oral thrush). Mycosis refers to any disease induced by fungus (of which yeasts are a subgroup). Mycotic vaginitis is generally assumed to be caused by Candida since Candida is the organism that causes the majority of vaginal and oral yeast infections. The terms *monilia* and *moniliasis* are also used for Candida, their usage dating from earlier this century after a series of taxonomic errors. Some practitioners, especially those in other countries, prefer to use them. Vaginitis is a general name for an irritation or inflammation of the vagina. Because over a dozen different culprits can be responsible for vaginitis, the term applies only to any generalized vaginal infection, unless it is clarified (e.g., bacteria vaginitis, trichomonal vaginitis, etc.).

Other names employed to describe vaginal yeast infections include: vaginal candidosis, candidal vulvovaginitis, chronic candidiasis, yeast vaginitis, vaginal moniliasis, monilial vaginitis, vulvovaginal candida, candidal, and yeast vulvovaginitis. All of these refer to the same condition: an infection in the vagina and vulva caused by a fungus of the genus *Candida.*

In addition to the terms used to describe a vaginal yeast infection, there are a variety of other medical terms used in this book that we define as we use them. If you do further reading, however, or even are just puzzled by jargon and medical terminology used by your doctor, we have provided a glossary of medical terms often used in the diagnosis and treatment of vaginal infections in Appendix A.

History of Yeast Infections

Yeast infections have plagued humankind since antiquity and consequently, the clinical manifestations of yeast infections have been noted by medical observers for centuries. Hippocrates, the father of medicine, described two cases of oral thrush in his treatise called *Epidemics,* published in the fourth century B.C. In both cases, he describes aphthae (white patches) in debilitated patients and associates the condition with severe underlying disease. Samuel Pepys, in his diary of June 17, 1665, writes: "He hath a fever, a thrush and a hickup [sic]."

Interest in fungal disease was substantial around the time of the American Revolution. Physicians and scientists around the globe found thrush a challenging and worthwhile research subject. In 1786 the French Société Royale de Médecine announced a sizable award for the study of thrush. It was not, though, until 1839 that the initial discovery was made of the organism that caused thrush; Langenbeck described a fungus and suggested it was the culprit that caused typhus. While his typhus theory turned out to be incorrect, his description of the fungus was nevertheless one of the earliest associations of such a microorganism with a pathological entity. Once the discovery of the thrush organism was made, mycologic medicine (the study of fungus in illness) proceeded at a much more rapid pace.

Thrush was recognized early on as a condition of the newborn, and Veron in 1835 postulated that it was acquired during passage through the womb. Five years later, Berg considered it to be transmitted by unhygienic conditions and communal feeding bottles. It was noted regularly as occurring in patients with debilitating diseases, confirming Hippocrates' original observations. Bennett, in 1844, and Robin, in 1853, both proposed that debilitation was the single most important precursor to candidal infection.

One of the first descriptions of vaginal candidosis was penned in 1849. J. Stuart Wilkinson wrote of a 77-year-old female patient with a profuse vaginal discharge. Quoting another doctor, Wilkinson said that he felt the "epiphytes" could not grow unless a "favorable soil was prepared for them." Previous to Wilkinson's observations, and for the next 40 years, vaginal discharge, as well as thrush, were defined in medical textbooks as a result of "morbid secretions."

The second half of the nineteenth century saw a marked increase in our understanding of yeasts. In 1875 Haussmann demonstrated that the causative organisms for both oral and vaginal thrush were the same. In contrast to the postmenopausal woman seeking help from Wilkinson, Mettenheimer, in 1882, described vaginal thrush in a virgin. In 1894 experimental inoculation of vaginal yeasts into rabbits was performed. The next year Herff reported his observations from studying over 13,000 hospital admissions: Candida infections were more common in warm climates than in cool ones.

While fungal diseases of all types were reported often in the latter half of the nineteenth century, they were little understood and often misdiagnosed. Marriage and childbirth were routinely held to blame for vaginitis and vaginal discharge (indeed, pregnancy was the event that triggered many cases of chronic vaginal thrush). It was not uncommon for cases of candidal vaginitis to be erroneously diagnosed as gonorrhea, an emotionally devastating mistake that continued into the early years of this century.

Over the years, research into mycotic infections has received considerable clinical and laboratory attention. *Candida albicans,* by far the predominant cause of thrush, has been scrutinized in fine detail by a variety of biochemists, microbiologists, and immunologists. While our knowledge of yeast infections, now at an all-time high, has led to the discovery of many antifungal formulations to combat the infections, the diseases caused by *Candida albicans* are nonetheless as common as ever.

The Incidence of Yeast Infections Is Rising Sharply

Vaginal yeast infections may have plagued our grandmothers and their grandmothers, but in absolute terms it is a far more common problem among women today. In spite of better hygiene, more understanding of our bodies, and an array of drugs effective against candidal infections, the growth in vaginal yeast infections has been dramatic since the 1960s.

Statistics on vaginal yeast infections in the United States are imprecise. Diseases considered to be transmitted sexually are monitored and tracked closely, but yeast infections are not included in this category. We do have estimates ranging from 20 to 50 million cases a year. American women purchased $220 million of prescription vaginal antifungal drugs in 1990.

Other countries keep much closer tabs on yeast infections. Genital candidosis is one of the most common fungal diseases in the United Kingdom. British researchers report that among women attending sexually transmitted disease clinics, yeast infections are the most common vaginal infection. British statistics show that the incidence is rising rapidly; between 1971 and 1981 the number of cases of candidal vaginitis rose by 42 percent. Australian researchers rank Candida as their most expensive gynecologic pathogen. In 1981 one million prescriptions for genital antifungals were filled in that country.

There are many reasons why cases of yeast vaginitis have mushroomed, but much of the rise can be linked with the beginning of widespread distribution and usage of two modern medical breakthroughs—antibiotics and birth control pills. Greater usage and availability of steroids and other immunosuppressant drugs have also made a contribution. Never has there been a time when so many women ingested so many antibiotics, hormones, and immunosuppressants. As we'll learn later, many of these prescription drugs alter the chemical makeup of the body and, in doing so, significantly reduce the body's natural yeast-fighting defenses. The more widespread usage of these drugs has become, the greater the incidence of yeast infections. In conventional medical wisdom, yeast infections are considered part of the fallout of living in the postantibiotic age.

Antibiotics, hormones, and immunosuppressants are not the only triggers of yeast infections. Lowered resistance to disease in general, pregnancy, poor hygiene, too much douching, vaginal cuts and/or abrasions, and sexual transmission have all been implicated.

We now find ourselves in a position where both the number of women suffering from yeast infections and the total number of yeast infections are at an all-time high. A woman under stress, rushing about frantically, eating more junk food than nutritious meals, taking antibiotics, and relying on birth control pills is a prime candidate for chronic candidal vaginitis. Unfortunately, it would seem that in this instance the modern conveniences and medical miracles of our society have left us more vulnerable to yeast infections than ever.

A Vicious Cycle

For the most part, yeast infections are considered relatively easy to treat. The woman with an occasional case of yeast vaginitis poses little therapeutic challenge in that a variety of home remedies or antifungals will generally clear up such an isolated infection conveniently and effectively. Women and their physicians, though, continue to be stumped by the problem of recurrent candidal vulvovaginal infection. Even using the most powerful prescription antifungal treatments, a significant percentage of women find themselves with a repeat infection shortly after eliminating or arresting the previous one.

There are over a half dozen specific topical antifungal drugs available today in a variety of formulations all designed to treat vaginal candidiasis. Primary cure rates (the percentage of women considered cured after completing the prescription) are generally in the 80–90 percent range. This is actually fairly low when you consider that we are dealing with a local treatment of a condition involving one single pathogen at an accessible site. But still, cure rates near 90 percent mean that almost everyone will find their infection cleared up after using the drugs with the remaining few almost always experiencing relief after a second course of treatment.

Studies have shown, though, that even if nine out of ten infections can be readily "cured," there is a real and constant problem with reinfection. In one study, conducted in the Netherlands, it was found that even though 96.3 percent of the women were cured after one week on antifungal therapy, the recurrence rate after four weeks was 26.9 percent. A study from Denmark reports relapse frequencies of up to 30 percent while yet another study in the U.S. reported that 71.4 percent of the participants had at least one repeat episode within six months after all were considered clinically cured.

One yeast infection can be a nuisance, but chronic yeast infections can be especially depressing. If you find yourself with infections often enough to consider them a problem, then you are already familiar with the daily inconveniences (pads to catch the discharge, cleansing often to contain the smell). Physical problems like painful sex and urination, and the irritation of the vulvovaginal area, coupled with the emotional toil of anticipating the discomfort and the lingering feeling that you are not being taken seriously by doctors, all make this a horrendous cycle. And on top of all that there is the expense of all those doctor visits, lab tests, and prescriptions. Once caught in the cycle of infection, the first sign of itching or discharge causes extreme distress. Your emotional health suffers as severely as your physical health.

Unless you read the medical literature, you may never realize just how common recurrence is. This is because the main source of drug efficacy information is through advertisements circulated by the pharmaceutical companies. In almost every study cited by the drug companies, the criteria are the same: results after completion of therapy (the cure rate) and results four weeks from treatment (the recurrence rate). The ads claim very high cure rates and very low recurrence rates. What the advertisements don't explain is that five weeks after treatments, two months after treatment, or six months after treatment the recurrence rates are still rising. Women who find themselves with repeat infections at more than four weeks and one day after using their medication are not counted in the statistics. So, while the actual percentage of recurrence can be as high as 75 percent, physicians and pharmacists are led to believe that the prescription antifungals are almost universally effective. This poses a real conflict at the doctor's when you report that the drugs are not working while the physician has every reason to believe the medications are completely adequate.

If our health care providers consider these "simple fungal infections" as relatively minor and the pharmaceuticals are so effective at curing them, why is it that yeast infections recur in so many women?

Where Do We Go from Here?

What do we know about vaginal yeast infections? We know that they affect women of all ages, but occur most frequently during the reproductive years. We know that a large percentage of these women have taken birth control pills and/or large doses of antibiotics. We know that there is often some factor that triggered the problem initially, but that even after that factor has been eliminated, the yeast infections may continue to come back. And we know that the medical community has disappointed a great many women in their inability to effectively diagnose and treat these infections, often dismissing them as either of minor medical importance or, in some cases, as a "normal part of being a woman."

In spite of the ubiquity and severity of recurrent vulvovaginal candidiasis, there has been no major change in the medical approach to the problem in decades. Whole journal issues devoted to yeast infections are striking in their lack of freshness. Research is focused more on comparing a five-day versus a seven-day course of treatment, rather than penetrating the unanswered question of recurrence. Pharmaceutical companies focus on the mere presence of yeast organisms as the culprit and that effective treatment necessitates the destruction of all yeast organisms in the vagina by using their products, of course. And most gynecologic textbooks still stress relief of symptoms and fail to emphasize the need to address the issue of recurrence.

The traditional remedies aren't working, and the newer antifungals are no better in the long term than antifungals available years ago. Yet these standard treatments generally focus on temporary relief and leave unaddressed the underlying factors triggering the problem.

New Hope—An Effective Treatment Program

Too many people go through an illness like this saying "Why is this happening to me?" instead of "What can I do about it?" Once I figured out that these repeat infections were an opportunity for me to take charge of my life, I was able to turn things around. I haven't had an infection for sixteen months now and I've never felt better!

—Social worker in Ann Arbor, MI

Only through increasing our knowledge of our bodies and of the yeast organisms with which we coexist can we begin to appreciate why the traditional remedies are inadequate. Understanding the nature of fungi and the mechanisms within our bodies to deal with them will help us understand the reason these infections continue to plague us.

The six chapters that follow review what is known in order to help you eradicate your yeast infections. Chapter 1 introduces you to the world of fungi and provides some insight into the organisms responsible for all the discomfort. Chapter 2 explains the factors that predispose your body to yeast infections. Chapter 3 dispels some of the myths surrounding these infections, explains the issues of self-diagnosis, and reviews other diseases which could be mistaken for yeast. Chapter 4 discusses when and why to seek medical attention, as well as reviewing some of the emotional turmoil you may have experienced. Chapters 5 and 6 cover treatment and prevention.

The book outlines a four-step approach to the successful treatment of vaginal candidiasis:

- Reduce the yeast population in your body
- Build up your beneficial bacterial population

- Limit and control your yeast triggers
- Strengthen your overall health

Following this four-step plan will make you a survivor rather than a victim of this scourge. By encouraging your body's natural yeast-fighting defenses with this program, you can soon look back on these infections as a chapter out of your past. Our goal in writing this book is to give women information and tools: information to understand some of the processes occurring in your body and tools to know when and how to respond. Knowledge is power, in this case the power to help heal yourself and take better care of yourself.

PART ONE

•

UNDERSTANDING YEAST

•

We never eat cookies because they have yeast,
And one little bite turns a man to a beast.
Can you imagine a greater disgrace,
Than a man in the gutter with crumbs on his face.

From "The Song of the Temperance Union"

1

🐌

ALL ABOUT FUNGI:
A Kingdom All Their Own

•

For years, all I ever heard was "We have to kill off the yeast, we have to kill off the yeast." I didn't really know much about this thing I was supposed to be killing so aggressively. Then this friend—he was a biologist—told me all about fungi. I don't want to kill them anymore. I have all this respect for the organism now.

—26-year-old long-distance runner

What do penicillin, the Irish potato famine, athlete's foot, Dutch elm disease, and soy sauce all have in common? Fungi. They would not exist were it not for fungi.

For hundreds of years botanists classified living things into two categories: the plant kingdom and the animal kingdom. Understandably, fungi were grouped in with the plants. However, as they became better understood—their complex breeding processes unraveled, their amazing ability to produce a multitude of chemicals analyzed, their incredible adaptability to wide and diverse environments appreciated—fungi earned an honor never before (or since) achieved: They were separated out of the plant group and put into a distinct group of their own. About two decades ago, botanists began classifying living things into three kingdoms: plant, animal, and fungus.

Fungi are not necessarily substances we think about or notice daily. Yet they touch our lives every day in many ways, for better and worse. They destroy tons of stored grain yet cure illnesses until only recently considered fatal. They are both key ingredients in the tool chest of biological warfare and gourmet foodstuffs sought after by trained pigs. Truly, they are amazing, contradictory organisms.

Fungi are extremely adaptable to diverse environments. Most grow best in moist warm climates, preferring temperatures between 70° and 90°F, and so tend to flourish in tropical lands. But they can easily survive being frozen for months or years at a time, which is why meat and other food must be stored below 20°F— to prevent them from molding. Similarly, molds (which are fungi) can grow in temperatures too hot for any warm-blooded creature, although they start to perish near 150°F and boiling (212°F) will finish off most of them instantly. Considering the range of temperatures in which fungi can sustain themselves, it is not surprising that they are found far and wide on this planet.

As children, many of us learned that animal life could not exist without green plants, the only living things able to convert energy from the sun into chemical energy (photosynthesis) which animals can then consume for nourishment. Yet if you back up one step, you'll see that most green plant life could not survive without the contributions of fungi. That is because fungi grow on and decompose the remains of plants and animals, converting them into rich soil. Without nutrient-rich earth, green plant life could not survive, which in turn, means that animals could not survive.

The primary task of fungus is to break down and recycle organic matter. Take a standard supermarket product: a box of crackers. Given the chance, fungi will consume the crackers, the plastic wrap which protects them, the box they are sold in, not even stopping to pause before devouring the glue and ink used in the packaging. Fungi are capable of decaying wood, cloth, fabrics, twine, electrical insulation, leather, keratin, fats, oils, phenols, asphalt, rubber tires, waxes, bones, foodstuffs, even the very microscope lenses from which we view them. In fact, given a sufficient amount of moisture, molding will begin within a week or two for practically all materials subject to fungal deterioration.

A whopping 100,000 species of fungi have been identified. While some are microscopic, 1/3,000 of an inch in diameter, others achieve sizes of over 70 inches in circumference and weights exceeding 300 pounds. Some have very limited diets, feeding, for instance, only on the left hind leg of a particular species of water beetle. Others consume just about anything, covering a range of materials so broad it is striking that our world has not become one gigantic mold colony.

Unlike plants, fungi do not have roots through which they can absorb water and nutrients. Instead, just like humans, they harbor chemicals which are responsible for digesting food. The basic notion of digestion is the same for both fungi and humans. Enzymes and acids work together to convert complex materials into simple ones. The essential difference between the human digestive system and that of fungi is that the fungi digest most of their foodstuffs outside their bodies. In other words, while humans eat first, then digest, fungi digest their foods before they eat them, breaking down complex substances, absorbing

them, and then converting the absorbed material into
more fungus.

Fungi, often considered simple organisms because
of their size are, in reality, extremely advanced forms of
life. They are very complex chemically, in fact producing a diversity of chemicals more varied and numerous
than any other life-form. In spite of their advanced
chemical prowess, all fungi, even a 100-pound puffball
mushroom, are considered "primitive" organisms; that
is, any single cell is capable of regrowing the entire
structure. If you thought of mosquitoes and cockroaches as prolific breeders, compared with many
fungi, insects aren't even in the competition. Take, for
example, a moldy orange. What you see as green dusty
mold is actually a penicillium colony (penicillin and
many other antibiotics are derived from a variety of
this mold). These spores cover the fruit like a thick
velvet blanket. The slightest disturbance of the fruit,
even just a ruffle of the air around it, sends up a cloud
of spores, millions strong, each cell capable of regrowing an entire colony.

So prolific are fungi that one single yeast cell, given
a highly favorable environment with a good assortment
of nutrients and the correct temperature, could produce a colony of over a hundred yeast cells within just
twenty-four hours. At this rate one individual cell,
within one week, could beget a yeast colony weighing
in at one billion tons. The fact is, though, that this does
not happen, and is not likely to happen, because the
environment is seldom ideal for any creature on earth,
yeast included.

The yeasts are microscopic single-celled organisms
which constitute one particular subgroup of fungi. The
single-celled, budding yeast is, in fact, the simplest
form of fungi. Yeasts are found around the world, especially abundant in sugary mediums, such as in flower
nectar and fruits.

An outstanding characteristic of many yeasts is their ability to convert sugar into carbon dioxide and alcohol, thus causing fermentation. One yeast cell can ferment approximately its own weight of glucose, the simplest form of sugar, per hour. The production of leavened bread, cheese, citric acid, beer, wine, vinegar, antibiotics, vitamins, and certain industrial compounds all depend on such fermentation.

This ability to cause fermentation is central to our appreciation of yeast. Indeed, in many languages the word for yeast derives from a description of what it does, rather than what it is: the French *levure* comes from the verb "to raise"; the German *hefe,* "to lift"; and the English word is derived from the Greek *zestos,* "boiled." The word *fermentation* itself is derived from the Latin, meaning "to boil" (the bubbling and foaming of fermenting liquids is visually similar to boiling). The fermentation caused by yeast is due to enzymes contained in the cells. Indeed, the word *enzyme* comes from the Greek words meaning "in yeast or leaven."

The antiquity of yeast is indicated by the discovery of these fungi in fossilized plants of the Devonian Age (340,000,000–405,000,000 years ago). Prescriptions containing yeast have been found in the Ebers Papyrus, one of the earliest known medical documents (sixteenth century B.C.). Hippocrates, the great Greek physician (fifth century B.C.) advocated yeast for certain diseases.

The extraordinary ability of yeast to cause fermentation brought it instant notoriety. Since many fermentative yeasts occur naturally on vegetable matter and in soil, alcohol no doubt originated accidentally. It wasn't long, though, before humans realized that if they carried over some of the active liquid from one brew to the next, they could have their alcohol and drink it, too. Brewing seems to have originated in Babylon where, as in Egypt, barley grew wild. There is some evidence that

beer made from malted grain was being brewed in
Mesopotamia as far back as 6000 B.C. In Egyptian
tombs of the eleventh dynasty (2000 B.C.) yeasts used
in the making of beer and bread have been found. A
brewer in California is attempting to reproduce a recipe
for beer translated from a 3,800-year-old stone tablet
with a hymn to Ninkasi, the goddess of beer in the
Sumerian civilization. In these earlier societies, beer
was enjoyed for its mood-altering qualities, as well as
enjoying an important role in religious worship and the
practice of medicine. In fact, although unaware of its
nutritional superiority, alcoholic beverages provided
early humans with more nutritional value than any
other food they had available, with the exception of
animal proteins. Some archaeologists and anthro-
pologists have even speculated that humans aban-
doned their hunting and gathering lifestyle for the
farming life in order to be able to maintain a steady
supply of alcoholic brew.

The raw materials of alcohol are carbohydrates and
yeast (potatoes and yeast produce vodka, grapes and
yeast produce wine). As grain and yeast were the keys
to producing beer, it was an obvious step for brewing to
be carried out by bakers. In fact, in the ancient world,
the twin arts of brewing and baking were inextricably
linked and considered of equal stature. These arts were
conducted in most large households from Mesopotamia until the early Middle Ages. As part of the
household chores, they remained largely the duty of
womenfolk. It was, ironically, the growth of monas-
teries, which used beer sales to generate income, that
resulted in both the development of large brewing units
and the transformation of the task to one dominated by
men.

While it is fungi that help cause the fermentation
which helps cause the leavening which creates a loaf of

bread, moldy bread (or, for that matter, meat, fruit, or milk) is undesirable, as yeast can spoil foods as well as create them. It is not always an obvious distinction. Some of the most delectable cheeses are ripened and given their characteristic flavors and textures by the same fungi that cause spoilage. Fungus grows, and partly digests (or rots) the milk curds and fat that will become, for instance, Roquefort cheese. It is the fungi that produce the bluish green substance distributed throughout the cheese in irregular veins and cavities. As Clyde Christensen, author of *The Molds and Man*, explains to the layperson, it sounds better to say that the cheese was softened and ripened by the mold, rather than to say it was partially rotted, but it is only a semantic difference.

Some of the same fungi that rot our foods also command high prices when they manifest themselves in the form of certain mushrooms. Whole industries have developed over the desire to add mushrooms to the mealtime palate, from dogs specially trained to sniff out difficult-to-find underground truffle patches to cottage industries producing gourmet oriental mushrooms in backyard manure ditches. We do not normally think of mushrooms as mold, yet there is little difference between common mold and common mushrooms. Both are fungi. Mushrooms just happen to be big enough to be seen, and tasty enough to be desired as food.

Yeast is also valuable as a food in and of itself. It is high in protein, as much as 50 percent by weight for dried yeast. It is rich in vitamins of the B group, including thiamine, riboflavin, and niacin, making it especially useful in the prevention and control of such food deficiency diseases as beriberi and pellagra. American brewers filter out most of the yeasts from beer, but the dark heavy British brews (chock full of yeasts replete with protein and vitamins) are still prescribed for the elderly in England to beef up their nutritional state.

It was Louis Pasteur, founder of the science of microbiology, who helped unravel some of the mysteries of fungi. The French scientist was the first to show that living things come only from other living things, disproving the then current notion of spontaneous generation. It was thought that fermentation either occurred spontaneously, the way maggots were thought to arise spontaneously from putrefied meat, or through some inorganic reaction similar to the oxidation of iron into rust. In 1857 Pasteur determined that the process of fermentation was actually a process brought about by feasting yeasts, and that each particular type of fermentation was the result of a specific microorganism acting on a specific type of substance to produce another substance.

At that time, the French wine industry was floundering from regular, but seemingly random, bitterness in the wine. Pasteur concluded that spoilage of such perishable products could be prevented by destroying the microbes present and protecting the then sterilized material against future contamination. Pasteur found that gently heating wine destroyed most of the microbes without altering the wine's flavor. By developing the heating process, Pasteur saved the wine industry (he had already saved the milk industry—but that's another story) and made his name a household word; to pasteurize is to use heat to partially sterilize liquids. Today, almost all milk, wine, and beer sold in the United States is pasteurized.

Just as Columbus didn't really discover America, Pasteur didn't really discover pasteurization. The Asians were actually way ahead. Soy sauce, sake, and cheeselike foods made from soybeans and rice were being manufactured with the aid of fungi in the Orient more than two thousand years ago. Before the Western world ever understood fermentation and wine production, the Japanese had developed the fermentation of sake to a fairly exact science. In fact, two hundred years before the time of Pasteur, Asians were heating finished wine to prevent later spoilage. As Clyde Christensen puts it in *The Molds and Man,* the Asians were "pasteurizing" their wine a couple of centuries before Pasteur was even conceived.

Nevertheless, we are greatly indebted to Pasteur for his contributions to medical science. Many of his contributions laid the groundwork for medical science as we know it. For instance, he not only found that each type of fermentation was caused by a particular type of germ, but also that each type of germ was responsible for a particular type of disease. This led him to one of the most fundamental facets in our medical knowledge—the germ theory of disease. Pasteur, in his effort to develop measures to minimize the spread of disease by microbes, developed the practice of using antiseptics. Additionally, after observing that birds which had been infected with old cultures of chicken cholera were resistant to the same infection, he founded the science of immunology and developed the first vaccine. Finally, in his pioneering work on rabies, he demonstrated that a disease could be caused by an agent so small it could not even be seen under a microscope, thus revealing the world of viruses.

Pasteur's work laid the foundation for the biggest breakthrough in the scientific world of fungus—the discovery of penicillin. In 1929 Dr. Fleming, working in a London hospital, noticed that a mold had contaminated a culture dish and inhibited the growth of bacteria. Ten years later a group of workers at Oxford, England, isolated the substance from the liquid in which this mold was grown. This substance, now known as penicillin, was capable of curing both mice and humans of what had been fatal infections caused by certain bacteria. Needless to say, the whole world of antibiotics was born.

While most people are somewhat aware of the tremendous benefits of penicillin and pasteurization, most are not versed in the many other claims to fame of fungi. The first hallucinogenic substances known to humans were fungi. Viking warriors of Scandinavia, consuming hallucinogenic mushrooms as far back as twelve centuries ago, enjoyed the invincible feeling it gave them as they terrorized and raided the British Isles. Ergot, a fungal disease of the rye plant, was responsible for many epidemics throughout Europe in the Middle Ages. It caused tremendous physical as well as mental illness, and insanity. In fact, lysergic acid, from which LSD is made, is also a fungal derivative.

Many fungi have been used for centuries as a healing medium, most commonly found in Chinese and Native American cultures. Certain fungi long suspected of having healing qualities have been shown scientifically to stimulate and strengthen the immune system; some are even known to exhibit anticancer agents. Also in the medical realm, a derivative of ergot has been used to stimulate uterine contractions in maternity practice.

There should not be anything surprising in the fact that we have been able to capitalize on the beneficial uses of a few fungi, such as penicillin. What is surprising is that of the tens of thousands of common fungi around us, we have been able to exploit only a dozen or so. And of those few, it turns out that every one was discovered completely by accident. Here we live in a world surrounded by hundreds of thousands of fungi, yet we remain largely ignorant of their powers and prowess.

Candida Albicans

There are more than 600 different kinds of yeasts. The yeast we are concerned with in this book is of the genus *Candida*. Although there are more than half a dozen species of Candida, the one of greatest importance in human infection is *Candida albicans*. While candidiasis can be a primary or secondary infection involving a member of the genus *Candida,* essentially the disease is an infection caused by the specific organism *Candida albicans.* Ninety-four percent of all cases of fungal vaginitis are due to *Candida albicans.*

Candida albicans makes its home in warm-blooded living beings all over the world; in fact, *C. albicans* does not routinely live in or multiply in nonanimal habitats. These yeasts reside throughout the body living on the mucous membranes. They thrive in warm, moist, dark recesses throughout the gastrointestinal tract (from mouth and nose to the esophagus, intestines, bowel, bladder, and anus) and in the vagina.

Candida organisms are not loners. They live in colonies along with vast quantities of bacteria also present throughout the gastrointestinal and vaginal tracts. In terms of sheer quantity, the yeast population is dwarfed by the bacterial population. This is no accident since one of the services the bacteria provide in your body is keeping the yeast population in check.

The fetus lives in a sterile environment. As long as the fetus remains secure in the womb, Candida is unknown to it. However, immediately upon exiting the womb, exposure to Candida often occurs during the passage out of the birth canal when the child swallows some of the mother's yeast-containing fluids. Failing that, the infant is nonetheless exposed almost immediately thereafter, either through inhaling yeast organisms in the air or through human contact. *C. albicans* often appears in the intestines of infants during the first week of life. However, its presence in the mouth, from whatever source, usually precedes the appearance of the organism in the intestinal tract.

Yeast is part of the makeup of a healthy body, where it is considered a commensal, an organism living in an intimate, nonparasitic relationship; it can also be present as a pathogen, capable of causing disease. Normally, Candida resides within animals harmlessly; indeed, its presence is entirely compatible with a lifetime of excellent health. It is equally apparent, however, that when there is ill health or physiological change, Candida can seize the opportunity and cause a remarkably wide range of infections.

The existence of Candida in its pathogenic state (as a disease) is seen primarily in humans. But it does affect other members of the animal kingdom, mainly birds like turkeys, parrots, hens, pigeons, fowls, and ducks. Other animals—hedgehogs, opossums, suckling pigs, and anteaters, as well as European and Indo-Chinese otters—have also been observed to get yeast infections.

Candida infections of almost every part of the body have been seen. Reports of skin and mucous membrane candidiasis greatly outweigh infections of other parts, but no organ has been spared infection by these microorganisms at some time. In its pathogenic state, Candida is responsible for a large number of distinctively different disease entities. In fact, Candida is recognized as one of the most frequently encountered fungal opportunists and is now regarded as the commonest cause of serious fungal disease.

Yeasts live in all of us, yet yeast infections only arise in individuals who become susceptible, either from a weakened state brought about by illness, by some other debility, or from a predisposing factor, as we will see in the next chapter. All people thus harbor within them an ecosystem of commensal yeasts which have a potential to become pathogenic.

The minimum daily requirements for yeast are minimal indeed—food, warmth, and moisture. Given these three conditions and a debilitated environment, the disease entities caused by Candida are many and varied. In fact, among infectious agents, only syphilis presents a clinical picture more diverse than that associated with the various candidiases. Among the persons affected are professionals whose occupations involve continual wetting of the hands, such as bartenders, dishwashers, fishmongers, and goosepluckers. A nail-biter can get paronychia (fungal infection of the nails); women get vaginal yeast infections; men, jock itch. Teenagers get athlete's foot. A denture-wearer can get oral thrush; a nursing mother, candida of the nipples; a baby, diaper rash.

Aside from skin infections, people can find themselves with internal disease, yeast infection of the bowel or an inflamed esophagus. Additionally, systemic or generalized infections of the lungs, liver, lymph nodes, spleen, and intestines may occur; these are occasionally fatal. Any drug (such as steroids) or disease (such as AIDS), that destroys the immune system accelerates the likelihood of such a systemic infection.

Fungal Infections in Perspective

It has only been in recent years that the significance of *Candida albicans* has come to be recognized in the field of medicine. Indeed, medical mycology, the study of fungus diseases, is relatively new. After all, a specific fungus could hardly be identified as a causal agent in an illness if it couldn't be recognized. It wasn't until medical science developed the ability to detect fungi in diseased tissue, isolate them, and prove by inoculation into laboratory animals that they were responsible for certain diseases, that the field of medical mycology began to evolve. The first human fungus was only described 100 years ago. Historically, most cases of Candida were diagnosed erroneously; yeast vaginitis was most commonly thought to be gonorrhea.

Today scientists have identified over four dozen fungal pathogens, a minuscule percentage of the roughly 100,000 species of fungi. Of these four dozen, twenty or so may cause widespread infection, twenty or so are regularly associated with skin infections, and another dozen or so are associated with severe, but localized subcutaneous (under the skin) disease.

Humans have an extremely high natural immunity to fungal diseases. With rare exceptions, the normal, healthy, well-nourished adult is resistant to all fungi, except in cases of overwhelming exposure. This means that fungus infections are almost entirely opportunistic, that is they become a disease-causing pathogen only when the situation and timing are right. The ability to cause infection, therefore, depends on either exposure to a sufficient amount of fungal organisms or to a state of generally reduced resistance in the body, or both.

Ironically, many of the triggers that contribute to the development of an infection are caused by or facilitated by recent medical breakthroughs (e.g., the Pill, antibiotics, immunosuppressant drugs, etc.). Altering the body by using these substances creates an ideal environment in which yeasts can thrive. Yeast infections, as a result, have increased in both number and severity as these drugs and treatments become increasingly pervasive. In actuality, yeast infections are simply the double-edged sword of miracle breakthroughs, as one expert in the field says: merely diseases of medical progress.

2

꿈

YEAST TRIGGERS

•

. . . symptoms in women with recurrent genital
candidosis were not caused by yeasts alone, and possibly the reason for recurrences might not lie in constant reinfection by yeasts, but in failure to recognize
and remove a primary underlying factor.

—Davidson/Mould,
British Journal of Venereal Diseases

What causes a yeast infection? No one knows exactly;
but we do know how yeasts behave and what factors
can trigger a yeast infection.

Yeast is ubiquitous. It is present in all living animals—it lives in our homes, in our houseplants; it is
present in many of the foods and beverages we consume. Indeed, yeast is all around us. Yet yeast infections do not plague all humans. The majority of people
on this planet live their entire lives without a single
yeast infection.

While we cannot point to one specific culprit and
declare it solely responsible for all the yeast infections
in the world, we have uncovered a body of evidence
that clearly shows how such infections can begin. Be-

fore we can understand the triggers of yeast infection
and our own susceptibility to them, we have to begin
with a simple premise: *Yeasts do not afflict healthy
individuals.* It is plain and simple. Since the yeasts are
already living in your body and in the environment all
around you, it is not a matter of an otherwise healthy
individual suddenly coming down with Candida (like
you can come down with the flu from an attacking
virus); rather, some altered physiological state must be
present in order for harmless yeasts to become
harmful.

Usually, we can apply a direct cause-and-effect
diagnosis to most bacterial or viral infections. The
doctor suspects an infectious agent, its presence is
verified by tests, direct observation, or corresponding
symptoms or other evidence. The bacteria or virus is
not supposed to be there; finding it indicates disease.
By the same token, its eradication eliminates the
disease. But yeast is different. Since yeast normally
lives in our bodies as a commensal (an organism which
lives in an intimate, nonparasitic relationship) determining that it has become a pathogen (an organism
capable of producing disease) and the specific how and
why of that transformation can be complicated. Nor is
it some Dr. Jekyll and Mr. Hyde transformation occurring within the yeasts. *Rather, it is a change in the host
(your body) that is necessary before Candida can induce its pathological effects.*

Natural immunity to fungal diseases is normally
very high. The healthy, well-nourished adult is resistant to almost all fungi, except in cases of overwhelming exposure (and with a handful of exceptions, such as
athlete's foot). Infection is dependent on some altered
state, and the existence of the infection indicates that
the body's natural defensive abilities are out of order.
Research has shown that it is not possible to induce
oral thrush in newborn lambs simply by putting the

fungi into their mouths; yet if they are weakened or debilitated in any way or if there is damage to the oral membranes, then thrush develops. Similarly, it has been a well-researched finding for decades that in pregnancy, women are more susceptible to Candida.

That candidiasis is not your everyday invasive disease is not a new discovery. Vaginal thrush was first described as a medical condition in 1849. Writings in the medical literature from the middle of the nineteenth century discuss the observation that thrush, local or widespread, occurs in those already weakened or stressed. In the second half of the 1800s, experiments were carried out in an attempt to verify these suspicions. In one study, a group of healthy women were vaginally inoculated with yeast organisms which had been taken from the vaginas of women who had active yeast infections. Symptoms of a yeast infection developed in a few of the women, yet in all cases, spontaneous cure occurred. Over a hundred years later, a similar experiment was conducted with the same result: spontaneous cure in all the participants. Experiments like these have been performed repeatedly, reaching the same conclusion: The vagina normally naturally rids itself of the disease, though the exact mechanisms for doing such are still unknown.

The conclusions of the nineteenth century physicians, working without benefit of our modern equipment or specialized training, were astute. Their observations are strikingly in accord with present-day views. As explained in the book *Candida Albicans,* the comments of the early researchers illustrate what appears to be the only valid generality with respect to yeast infections. In 1869 Trousseau, summarizing 25 years of research papers, described the disease as *the local expression of a very bad state of the whole system.* In 1877 Parrot, another physician, wrote that *thrush is a disease of the diseased.* Bennett of Edinburgh felt it probable that fungus always arose in living animals previously diseased and that their presence was indicative of *great depression of the vital powers and impairment of the nutritive functions*. Debilitation, they all concluded, was the most important prelude to candidal infection.

Many physicians miss this point, that the yeasts are secondary invaders simply seizing an opportunity brought about by a compromised state of health. They treat the yeast infection without establishing if there may be any underlying causes, incorrectly assuming that the mere presence of yeast is the cause of disease. This incorrect assumption is one reason why so many women are sent home with prescriptions for costly pharmaceuticals after a brief description of symptoms or routine exam indicating the presence of yeast. *Neither the presence of yeasts nor the quantity of yeasts is an accurate indicator of infection*. One study reported in a 1978 *British Journal of Venereal Diseases* found a complete dissociation between symptoms and yeast population. The researchers concluded that Candida is always a secondary invader in the vagina, either combining with an underlying factor to produce symptoms or enhancing the symptoms the primary factor has already produced. In fact, the extent and severity of the disease usually correlates with the severity of the underlying illness.

Accepting that yeast can be present without symptoms of vaginitis and that healthy women possess a natural ability to rid themselves of this condition means that we need to make a radical departure from the standard medical approach to curing yeast infections. Health professionals, treating yeast vaginitis, focus treatment on eradicating the fungus, not trying to elicit the cause. Prescriptions are employed to kill the yeast, which, however, provide little more than short-lived symptomatic relief. There are, fortunately, an in-creasing number of medical providers who will work with the patient to uncover and remove any and all underlying factors acting as yeast triggers. The road to recovery has less to do with eliminating yeast than with improving the vigor of the human.

If Candida is never the primary invader but simply an opportunistic organism taking advantage of an otherwise debilitated environment, the obvious ques-tion to ask is what debilities encourage yeast to be-come pathological. Major illnesses, such as mononucle-osis or strep throat can obviously leave you weakened (not to mention pumped full of antibiotics) and there-fore susceptible to a yeast infection. But yeasts are highly opportunistic and do not require anything as dramatic or extreme. Any condition that leaves you in less than optimal health can allow a yeast problem to get started. The yeasts may grow wildly, causing an infection almost immediately or grow slowly over time, with symptoms mild enough to ignore for a time. Once they become entrenched in your body, however, the yeasts are not eager to relinquish control.

Studies analyzing both the behavior of yeasts and case studies of women with recurrent yeast vaginitis have consistently found a handful of factors that trigger yeast production and susceptibility. The primary trig-gers, generally recognized as predisposing conditions, are:

- Antibiotic Therapy
- Oral Contraceptives
- Poor Menstrual Management
- Pregnancy, Childbirth, and Breast-feeding
- Sexual Transmission
- Genital Abrasion/Irritations
- Immunosuppressant Therapy

- Other Weaknesses in Immune System:
  Poor Nutrition, Stress, Illness
- (Infancy)

Any debilitating illness or any of the above conditions, individually, but especially in combination, are prime invitations for yeast infection. The severity and extent of Candida infections increases with both the number and severity of these predisposing conditions. Being aware of some of the common yeast triggers will enable you to avoid them, where possible, or react to them with appropriate measures to counteract their yeast-enhancing effects. This chapter will look at each of these separately and examine how each affects yeasts in your body.

Antibiotic Therapy

You mention the word *penicillin* to me and I get a yeast infection.

—24-year-old stockbroker

I'll never forget this one particularly bad time in college. I had this really bad throat infection and was on high doses of antibiotics. I can remember it so clearly—my throat was killing me and my crotch was, too.

—29-year-old in Ithaca

Antibiotics have eliminated or controlled so many infectious diseases that almost everyone has benefited from their use at one time or another. The other side of the coin, though, is that doses of antibiotics over the years have more than likely contributed to your yeast problem in a significant way. Many women are familiar with the reality that a yeast infection often follows a course of antibiotics. The increased incidence of candidiasis in recent years is clearly related to the increased use of antibiotics with research showing as much as a tenfold increase in candida vulvovaginitis in patients using antibiotics. "Not only are antibiotics responsible for the increased frequency with which women are colonized with Candida today," says Dr. J. D. Sobel, "but antibiotics are probably the most commonly identified precipitating factor of vaginitis."

Antibiotics encourage yeast growth in several ways, primarily by killing off the bacterial organisms in the body. This accomplishes the goal of killing off the offending organisms responsible for, say, bladder infections, tonsillitis, or sinusitis. Unfortunately, antibiotics are not so finely tuned that they eliminate just the offending bacteria. They also kill off "good" bacteria that have been working to retain and control the internal yeast population. The absence of bacteria alters the environment so that existing *Candida albicans* organisms are given an opportunity to reproduce and colonize unrestricted.

Antibiotic use, for the woman prone to yeast infections, is asking for a triple whammy. First, the antibiotics kill off bacteria that help keep the yeast population in check. Second, there is evidence that antibiotics, particularly those in the tetracycline group, may themselves actually stimulate yeast growth. Third, it appears that one effect of antibiotics is to alter the bodily tissue in such a way as to admit fungal organisms more easily.

In addition, it is impossible to separate the effects of the antibiotics, per se, from the effects of the illness that led to their use. Since yeast does not attack healthy individuals, the presence of an illness that warrants antibiotic use at all means that the yeast infections are more likely to occur anyway.

Many doctors routinely prescribe for yeast-prone

women an intravaginal antifungal medication whenever an antibiotic is recommended hoping that this will counter the effects of the antibiotic on the vaginal yeast population. It is not known how effective this is, but in many cases, it does work. However, for women who have other predisposing conditions, have had long-term treatment with antibiotics, or who have had multiple courses every year for years, it may not be enough. Each time antibiotics are taken, the internal ratio between bacteria and yeast gets thrown out of whack. If this is minor, corrective action may not be required. But a small imbalance multiplied over time could leave you with a serious yeast problem where corrective action (versus preventative action) is the only solution to solving the intractable yeast infections.

Many women who, as adults, find themselves with chronic yeast vaginitis have taken repeated courses of antibiotics. Extended antibiotic use in treating children and adolescents is common; many kids take antibiotics for years and years as a treatment for ear infections and acne.

Readers will find practical suggestions, including information on concomitant antifungal therapy, for those times when antibiotics are wanted or needed, as well as information on the side effects from antibiotic use, in the "Guide to Taking Antibiotics" at the end of chapter 6. Additional information can also be found in Appendix B, which lists the drug and brand names of broad- and narrow-spectrum antibiotics.

Another Source of Antibiotics

Swallowing antibiotic tablets in the form of prescription drugs is not the only way we end up consuming them. Half of all the antibiotics produced in this country are fed to livestock as grain additives. When antibiotics are fed to poultry and farm animals, they can grow up to 20 percent heavier. Not only do the antibiotics (along with additional hormones added to the feed) increase the amount of growth, they also increase their rate of growth so the animals get bigger faster (which makes it easy to see why farmers do it). Additionally, these substances help control farm animals' susceptibility to disease that their unnatural existence generates. Almost all commercially produced meat and poultry in the United States (70 percent of cattle and almost all pigs and fowl) comes from farm animals given such a diet.

Remember that truism: You are what you eat? It turns out that organisms (including antibiotics, hormones, and disease-causing entities) within animals find their way into the human intestinal tract when the animals are consumed. How prevalent is human ingestion of antibiotics through animal products? Penicillin can be found in almost every quart of commercially produced milk and anyone who regularly eats beef, pork, veal, and poultry has absorbed prodigious amounts of antibiotic and hormonal residues. The only way to avoid this is to eat meat raised on farms that do not use such supplementation or to consume a diet high in lamb or seafood (which can be an expensive dietary change). Intake of these drugs over many years may have an effect on the body's immune system; however, very little data exists on this subject.

Anyone who has problems with yeast should avoid taking antibiotics as prescription drugs whenever possible, and try as well to reduce their consumption of high amounts of commercially raised meat. Fish, lamb, and/or meat raised free of antibiotics and hormones (available in health food stores and some supermarkets) are sources of animal protein without this added complication, as are all the staples of a vegetarian diet.

(The antibiotic source in meat should be especially noted by followers of the yeast-free diet, a regimen high in protein and low in carbohydrates. As a diet high in animal protein may also be a diet high in antibiotics, practitioners of the yeast-free diet may inadvertently be consuming antibiotics—which are also supposed to be avoided. [Chapters 3 and 6 have more information on the yeast-free diet.])

Oral Contraceptives

There is . . . little doubt amongst those who have been in venereology for thirty years that the advent of the contraceptive pill, halfway through the period, has been associated with a profound change in the incidence of vaginal candidiasis . . .

—Drs. Morton and Rashid,
Proceedings of the Royal Society of Medicine

The contraceptive pill is the most common form of birth control used in America today. As many as 9 million women use this form of birth control. Many women have been taking contraceptive hormones for decades, starting in their adolescent years and continuing through their twenties and thirties. It is not uncommon for girls to start taking the Pill years before becoming sexually active since it is often prescribed to alleviate acne and regulate the menstrual cycle as well as to prevent undesired pregnancies. Though the Pill ushered in new freedom for women, it also engendered a significant increase in the number of women finding themselves with yeast infections.

Research over the past 25 years has consistently found that women who use oral contraceptives are significantly more likely to suffer from vaginal candidiasis. Studies throughout the 1970s and '80s confirmed the results of "Pill-associated" vaginitis even with the lower dosage pills now available. A 1985 study reported increases in candidiasis of nearly 80 percent among women using the Pill; oral contraceptives were cited as the causative factor in 50 percent of the cases of vaginal candidiasis in a 1984 article; and another study showed a significant correlation between Pill use and the occurrence of yeast vaginitis. Whether the exact percentage is 50 percent or 80 percent, for women prone to yeast infections, oral contraceptives may be a significant contributor to the problem.

The main reason for this is that the Pill, simply put, works by inducing hormonal changes that correspond closely to those of pregnancy. Since a female human does not continue to conceive once conception has occurred, the Pill's effectiveness is derived from its ability to simulate pregnancy. By tricking the body into thinking it is pregnant, actual conception does not occur. The catch: Pregnancy is a major predisposing factor for yeast infections. In fact, one or multiple pregnancies often triggers the cycle of infection. Long-term Pill use simulates in your body some of these effects of pregnancy, thus creating the predisposition to yeast infection.

The female body produces the hormone estrogen throughout the monthly cycle. Progesterone, another hormone, is produced at ovulation, preparing the lining of the uterus for the release and attachment of the egg. Throughout pregnancy, the body maintains a high level of progesterone. Both estrogen and progesterone are present in varying proportions in most birth-control pills, and any woman using them will have much higher levels of progesterone than a nonpregnant, non-Pill user. For reasons we don't yet understand, progesterone greatly aggravates yeast growth in women.

The Pill alters both the content and acidity (pH) of the vagina. One of the ways we have of monitoring the vaginal environment is by measuring how acidic or alkaline it is. The pH scale is a numeric measuring system with ranges from 1 to 14. Measurements between 7 and 0 represent increasing degrees of acidity, measurements above 7 represent increasing degrees of alkalinity (or basicity), and 7.0 is neutral. The healthy vagina normally maintains itself at levels between 3.8 and 4.2 without intervention. To give you an idea of the pH system, vinegar, wine, and orange juice all measure less than 4.0, saliva is 5.5, milk is 7.0. The pH of the vagina among Pill users rises to as high as 6.5. This makes the internal vaginal environment less acidic and more unstable than desirable (unless you happen to be a yeast organism).

Oral contraceptive users also have a much "sweeter" vagina, literally. The glucose (or sugar) content of the vaginal environment is increased by up to 80 percent in comparison with normal. The vaginal mucous membranes are also altered in such a way that allows yeasts to multiply more easily. Nursing women taking oral contraceptives with low estrogen content may also be more susceptible.

In Pill users as in pregnant women, once a yeast infection is established, it is harder to eradicate. In fact, women taking the Pill often require double or triple the antifungal prescriptions in order to clear up the infection, and in some cases, the Pill must be discontinued before a cure can be achieved. For all the convenience and freedom the Pill affords, those benefits are reduced significantly for that percentage of Pill users who find themselves trading convenience and freedom for discomfort and distress. Not all Pill users suffer from yeast infection, but the numbers are significant enough and the evidence strong enough to justify discontinuation of the Pill if such infections do begin to make repeat appearances.

The section "Getting Off the Pill," in chapter 6,

provides more information and suggestions for women using oral contraceptives.

Poor Menstrual Management

When I was younger, I'd enjoy getting my period. But in my midtwenties, I started getting yeast infections, first fairly randomly, then increasingly, but always right at the time of menstruation. I really began to dread getting my period. But now I know all these little tricks, like cutting down on sweets, taking acidophilus, and doing vinegar douches, that keep the infections at bay. Not only do I like getting my period again, but I especially like knowing that by taking care of myself, I can keep routine problems at bay.

—32-year-old from St. Louis

A woman's body goes through a series of changes each month around the time of menstruation. Most of the changes directly or indirectly encourage yeast growth, making one week in four a potential danger zone for infection. Significant changes in hormone levels coupled with an environment where warm blood is present 24 hours a day makes this time of the month particularly conducive for yeasts.

Just before menstruation, estrogen and progesterone levels reach their peak. These hormones greatly aggravate yeast growth in the same way they aggravate yeast growth in pregnancy when they are at similar levels. Centuries of clinical observation have taught us that vaginal candidiasis is influenced by women's hormone cycles, with more occurrences premenstrually (and late in pregnancy) when these estrogen and progesterone levels are at their highest.

Another effect of the hormonal changes are the symptoms women experience, to different degrees, before and during menstruation. These include fatigue, irritability, cravings for sweets or specific foods, cramps, back pain, headaches, and more. The net result of these menstrual reactions is that some women find themselves more stressed, more fatigued, and more likely to be consuming nutritionally poor food prior to, and during, menses. All of these—stress, fatigue, and nutritional imbalance appear to contribute to your yeast susceptibility.

The mere presence of blood during menstruation has surprisingly positive effects on the yeast population. The first thing that the presence of blood affects is the vaginal pH with the normally stable, acidic vagina turning alkaline since menstrual blood (as is all blood) is alkaline. This natural altering of the local environment means that a normally stable ecosystem is thrown out of kilter, making you susceptible to opportunistic situations of all kinds. (Sexual excitement and semen also raise the pH of the vagina, so that sexual activity during menstruation can raise the vaginal pH even more significantly.)

Another way that blood encourages yeast growth is by providing the yeast with an abundant food supply. While menstrual blood may seem like a messy nuisance to a human, it is a boon for yeast, a nutrient-rich food source that the yeast can actually use to grow, multiplying quickly and in vast numbers.

Finally, menstrual blood is warm and moist, two conditions necessary to the survival of yeasts. When you wear a sanitary napkin, you close off the warm moist vagina with its built-in food source, and you actually encourage rapid yeast growth. Women who use tampons, conversely, find themselves with yeast infections less frequently. It appears that allowing the vagina to air out and dry, by using tampons instead of pads, and washing and letting yourself air dry, diminishes the comfort of the yeasts' home.

Hormonal fluctuations, PMS and menstrual stress, fatigue and poor nutrition, an altered alkaline pH, and a warm, damp, nutrient-rich ecosystem—all provide the perfect combination for regular yeast infection. Since each month brings a period of high susceptibility, any measures you can integrate into your monthly habits which may counter these yeast-encouraging trends will make a difference. See chapter 6 for specific advice on ways to manage your cycle to combat yeast.

Pregnancy, Childbirth, and Breast-feeding

Candidal vaginitis is the most frequent of all infections in maternity practice. . . . Treatment during pregnancy is often neglected, or stinted, and is by no means so successful as the claims of manufacturers or the earlier literature indicated. A retrospective survey of some five hundred women treated for pregnancy thrush showed that 45 percent had had more than one course of treatment during pregnancy, and one luckless woman had had nine courses. This does not tally with the 85–95 percent cure rates claimed . . .

—Dr. Rosalinde Hurley, 1976

At one point last year, I decided to find a female gynecologist, hoping she would be more understanding than the male doctors I had seen. When I complained to her about my repeated yeast infections, her response was short and not-so-sweet: "Honey, you think you've got it bad now, just wait until you're pregnant."

—25-year-old editor in Chicago

For centuries, vaginitis and vaginal discharge were thought to result from marriage and childbirth (which often went hand in hand). This association makes some sense since pregnancy vaginitis seems to be the triggering event in many cases of vaginal thrush. In fact, fungal vulvovaginitis is the most common of all the infectious diseases of pregnancy.

As we know, the yeast organism is frequently found in the vagina. While approximately 15 percent of nonpregnant women harbor Candida in the vagina, the percentage is tripled among pregnant women. To make matters worse, the population of vaginal yeasts continually increases in pregnant women throughout the 40 weeks of pregnancy. With this increase in vaginal yeast organisms often comes vaginal yeast infection with the incidence of vaginal candidiasis climbing as the pregnancy continues so that over 50 percent of women in their final trimester are affected.

> There is nothing like a yeast infection when you're pregnant. My girlfriend and I used to refer to them as our "cheese factories." It got so bad, we had to learn to joke about it just to save our sanity.
>
> —29-year-old chemist in Syracuse

A 1984 study involving 600 women found that pregnancy was the most likely precipitator of yeast vaginitis. Why is pregnancy such a significant precursor to yeast infection? There are a number of suspected reasons, many of them similar to what we have seen with yeast and the Pill. The high levels of estrogen and progesterone associated with pregnancy directly encourage yeast colonization, not only making you more likely to have an infection when you're pregnant, but also making it harder to treat the condition. In fact, cure rates are significantly lower during pregnancy.

Additionally, the high levels of estrogen during pregnancy result in an abundance of glycogen (sugar) in the vaginal mucous membranes. This provides the yeast with an abundant, nourishing food supply. Pregnancy also raises the vaginal pH significantly and affects the vaginal tissues, two events that can promote yeast infections.

Over half of all pregnant women spend their third trimester dealing with yeast infections which can produce an abundant white, cheesy discharge that leaves the vagina almost constantly wet. The frequent need to urinate compounds the itching and irritation. The final three months of pregnancy are just about the last time women should have to be saddled with yeast infections.

Of course, pregnancy usually ends with childbirth and the good news is that soon after the birth the vaginal yeast population rapidly declines. The bad news is that tears and abrasions from the birth also provide a great environment for yeast, fueled by the almost constant presence of blood for weeks afterward. Unfortunately, though, the end of the pregnancy does not always signal the end of the yeast infections. For some, the cycle of yeast infections that had established itself during pregnancy continues.

The healthy pregnant woman has greater caloric needs than her nonpregnant counterpart. In addition, she needs greater amounts of protein and higher levels of certain nutrients (most notably iron, calcium, and folic acid). Part of the miracle of pregnancy is that even if the mother's diet is inadequate, nature tries to protect the developing fetus from malnutrition by supplying it with nutrients—at the expense of the mother. Maintaining good health during and after pregnancy can be challenging especially if the mother is under stress, maintaining a busy schedule, experiencing morning sickness or generally feeling poorly, or is too uncomfortable to get all the rest her body requires.

Breast-feeding is the new mother's way of providing her child with optimal nutrition and the closest bonding. Nursing mothers require extra calories, protein, and calcium, as well as extra iron to replenish what was lost through bleeding in delivery. A varied and balanced diet, and all the household help you can get are certainly in order to ensure that you can provide the new baby with the very best and take care of yourself, too.

In addition to the special nutritional demands, new mothers are the only category of women in their reproductive years who may find themselves with atrophic vaginitis, a condition due wholly or in part to a lack of estrogen. Vaginal pH may rise as high as 7.0. Symptoms may include vaginal soreness and occasional spotting. There may be itching and a watery discharge, and intercourse may be painful. During atrophic vaginitis, the vaginal walls become thinner and more susceptible to infection. Health professionals usually treat this condition with vaginal lubricants, and topical or oral estrogen.

Given the demands of pregnancy, childbirth, and breast-feeding, it is not hard to see how a woman could give birth to a healthy baby, but then enter motherhood exhausted. Sleepless nights, emotional and/or financial stress, shifting hormones, and high nutritional requirements all await the new mother. Additionally, tears, abrasion, and blood around the vagina invite growing yeast organisms. Multiple pregnancies, especially if closely spaced, may also magnify the situation.

Tips on treatment and prevention of yeast vaginitis during pregnancy—and after—can be found in chapter 5.

Sexual Transmission

Candida vaginitis can be a venereal disease, since it can be transmitted from partner to partner by sexual activity. The male may harbor Candida on or around his genitals and introduce the fungus into the female at the time of sexual intercourse. Likewise, the male may contract Candida from an infected partner. Some cases of recurrent Candida vaginitis occur because the infected sexual partner has not been treated.

—Wunderlich/Kalita, *Candida Albicans*

The issue of whether candida infections can be triggered from sexual transmissibility is steeped in as much emotion as science. Some find it inexcusable and indefensible not to examine and treat both (or all) sexual partners, especially in the instances of recurrent vaginitis. Unfortunately, opinion seems divided, but many doctors feel that a male has no role in the condition whatsoever, that it is entirely a woman's problem. It is, however, interesting to note that the Centers for Disease Control classifies candidal vaginitis as a venereal disease.

When we consider the sexual transmissibility of Candida, there are four areas that need attention and discussion. Can you get a yeast infection from oral sex? Can you get a yeast infection from heterosexual intercourse? Can you get a yeast infection from anal intercourse? Can you get a yeast infection from lesbian sexual activities? The issue of heterosexual transmission is the only issue addressed in the medical literature and the only one for which studies have been performed. Therefore, the bulk of this section will deal with findings on transmission through male/female vaginal intercourse. However, these will allow us to draw some conclusions about oral, anal, and lesbian sex, all discussed at the end of this section.

The possibility that yeast infections could be passed to a partner or passed back and forth between partners is not revolutionary thought. Thrush passed between wet nurses and infants has been observed for over a century. Sometimes a mother or caretaker and an infant can get into such a bad cycle of transmitting thrush to each other that the adult will have to wear rubber gloves for a few days in order to break the infection. Unsterilized pacifiers, bottles, and diapers have also been implicated as culprits in transference of fungal infections. Since these types of infections are from the same Candida organism that causes vaginal yeast infections, this suggests that sexual transmission is a real possibility.

Doctors are beginning to consider and treat the partner when a sexually active woman suffers from recurrent vaginitis. Some health professionals will concede that an uncircumcised male could possibly be harboring the yeast organism, but in fact, a man does not require a foreskin in order to harbor Candida. The organism has been found in the urethra, in the small grooves on the penile cap, and in the penile fluids (as well as the digestive and urinary tracts) as easily as in any narrow crevices created by a foreskin.

The first articles on candidiasis of the penis and surrounding skin, usually in the husbands of women with vaginal thrush appeared in the medical literature in the 1920s. Today, over 15 percent of the patients surveyed about connections of sexual intercourse to Candida infections report a positive history of such occurrences, with affected women reporting subsequent infection of their partners and vice versa. One research team found that, statistically, yeasts were probably spread by sexual transmission in 30–40 percent of all cases of genital candidiasis.

The nurse practitioner in college told me that some guys come in for jock itch; they've tried using the correct products, unsuccessfully. What they really had is exposure to yeast from women. At the health clinic, if you had a yeast infection, the nurses always sent you home with sample tubes of Monistat for the boyfriends to use.

—Student in Wisconsin

Studies comparing yeast infections to method of contraception show that people who do not use any form of birth control have fewer yeast infections. One conclusion which could be drawn from this is that women who do experience yeast candidiasis are more likely to be using some method of contraception. Another conclusion is that people who are sexually active are more likely to get yeast infections. Since people who use no birth control are typically not engaging in sexual activity, and people who use birth control get more yeast infections, many researchers draw the conclusion that sexual transmission is a factor.

Sometimes my husband gets a real bad itch the night we have intercourse or the morning after. With the itching, he gets irritation and dry patches. We've learned that when he gets that itching, I am just about to get another yeast infection. I am convinced that we pass the yeast back and forth. As soon as the itching on him begins, we both start with Monistat and vinegar rinses.

—32-year-old illustrator

The evidence that men may play a role in women's yeast infections is significant. Dr. Sobel reported in 1985 that male sexual partners of women with yeast infections are four times more likely to have penile colonization than men whose partners are not infected. "About eighty percent of female contacts of infected men have positive yeast cultures versus only thirty-two percent of women with uninfected partners. Typing the strains from both partners reveals that in the majority of cases both members harbor the identical strain. . . ." Further studies support this hypothesis, establishing that the ejaculate of husbands of women with the recurrent disease often yields Candida species, that seminal fluid contains agents that promote yeast growth, and that the yeast strain detected in the mouth, intestinal tract, or genital tract of a woman was always identical to that found in the genital tract of her male partner.

Leading researchers agree that the sexual partner(s) should always be treated in any situation where a sexually active woman is suffering from recurrent yeast vaginitis. One standard medical text, *Harrison's Principles of Internal Medicine*, states: *Unless the sexual partner is treated when candidiasis is present, there will be a constant retransfer of the infection.* By treating a partner harboring yeast, you remove a predisposing factor of vaginitis and are that much closer to breaking the cycle of infection, especially for sexually active women with recurrent infection.

The emphasis of this book is on women suffering with candidal infection, but men may also experience symptoms of candidal infection, usually referred to as Candida balanitis and/or Candida balanoposthitis. These symptoms may include some or all of the following: penile reddening; dryness; itching; inflamed, weeping mucosal surfaces of the glans penis and the prepuce; and bright red spots around the penis, sometimes covered with white membranes.

> I've had problems with three different male lovers in transferring yeast infections. There was one in particular I felt real bad about. I think he suffered more from my yeast infections than I did.
>
> —24-year-old stockbroker

Candidiasis of the penis, while admittedly not as prevalent as vaginal candidiasis, has attracted very little research interest. In addition to an actual case of a penile fungal invasion, some men have an allergic reaction on the genitalia after exposure to yeast. Happily, the allergic condition disappears when the partner is treated and her vaginitis cured.

Male partners of women with vaginitis may not be harboring yeast, may be asymptomatic carriers of the fungus, or may have symptoms and/or pain. In cases

---

In discussing the issue of male colonization of Candida, there are actually two issues that need to be addressed. The first, of course, is potential reinfection of the female. The second issue is any infection or discomfort the male may experience as a result of engaging in intercourse with his partner.

Advocates of the "It's a woman's problem" school of thought point to a handful of articles that "prove" that treating the male has no effect. One typical study (performed in The Netherlands and Belgium) is repeatedly cited as proof that treating a male partner has no effect on the incidence of vaginitis in the female. The researchers concluded that cure and recurrence rates did not differ when the sexual partner was treated. Their treatment for both women and men consisted of oral ketoconazole (in varying doses) taken for a total of three days. Recurrence rates for the women ranging from 27 percent to over 56 percent were reported. This study and others like it only prove that the prescribed treatment is hardly a satisfactory one; such strikingly high recurrence results, regardless of whether the partner took the treatment or the placebo, are not convincing on the question of partner cotreatment. The only conclusion which should be drawn from such research is that a three-day regimen of ketoconazole is hardly an effective treatment approach for anyone.

where recurrence is an issue, treatment of the partner is appropriate. Mutual genital infection in sexual partners, via the vagina-penis-vagina route, may be an important source of reinfection in cases of chronic Candida vaginitis.

Sexual Transmissibility: Oral, Anal, and Lesbian Sex

There is little research or discussion in the medical literature of sexual transmission other than through heterosexual vaginal intercourse. Many people ask whether yeast infections could be spread through oral or anal sex. Lesbian women also find themselves wondering if yeast infections can be spread among partners. None of the popular books on women's health discusses these topics, and women may not feel comfortable enough or confident enough with their physicians to ask.

Transmission through anal intercourse is definitely possible. Yeasts are prevalent in the bowel; in fact, the bowel, as part of the gastrointestinal tract throughout which these organisms live and reproduce, generally harbors the largest yeast colonies in your body—three to four times that of the vagina. Transfer of yeasts from the anal region to the vagina has been reported, and is the suspected culprit in many cases of vaginal candidiasis. Women struggling with yeast vaginitis should avoid any activities that would allow organisms to be moved from the anus to the vagina. For example, you should avoid inserting anything (penis, vibrator, fingers, etc.) into the vagina that has had contact with an anus—it could result in a high level of exposure and therefore a massive effort for your body to then reduce the vaginal yeast population back to normal.

Passing the infection back and forth between women from mouth or fingers to the vagina seems possible, but the likelihood is slight. There is no good evidence that yeasts actually get transferred this way, although it is always a good idea to avoid putting anything into the vagina if it has been in the anus. Remember, too, the issue is not the presence of yeast, but the body's ability to respond to it. Simple exposure to yeast is not sufficient to cause someone to develop an infection. There must be a combination of exposure to yeast with a lack in the body's ability to ward off the infection.

The bottom line is that there is very little research in the areas or oral or anal transmission. There is only one study that even mentions the possibility of transmission through oral sex and it has no definitive conclusions. Similarly, in dental literature, little has been published on the transmissibility of oral thrush through kissing. Sexual transmission studies always assume heterosexuality. The lack of medical data in these two areas may indicate lack of interest in such studies, but more than likely indicates that there is little suspicion of any connection. None of the lesbian couples interviewed in conjunction with the research for this book suspected they had been transmitting yeast through intimate sexual contact.

Though oral/vaginal transmission does not appear to pose a large risk, there is no reason not to take basic preventative measures. The primary prevention technique is, of course, the obvious one: maintain a good state of health. If you are healthy, the yeasts are unlikely to trouble you. Other prevention techniques have been advocated, but there is no clinical data to support or refute them. Suggestions include: over-the-counter antifungal mouthwash, such as Orithrush from Ecological Formulas (8 ounces sell for $12.95), that can be used before oral sex if you want to minimize exposure to yeast; using Nystatin powder mixed with a little water to make an antifungal mouth rinse (grape or grapefruit juice mask the taste well); and using mouth-washes as douches if you want to minimize a partner's exposure to any yeast from the genitalia.

For more information on treating the partner and minimizing the risks of sexual transmission see chapter 5.

Genital Abrasions/Irritations

Normally, I don't have a lot of trouble with yeast infections, but I have to take precautions. I've learned the hard way that there are certain things that will really irritate my vagina, and when that happens, I inevitably get a yeast infection. There are some spermicides I just can't use, and the contraceptive sponge will do it every time.

—24-year-old in Arizona

Numerous experiments have been conducted where a clinician attempts to create a yeast infection in a willing volunteer. Aside from the attempts at inducing vaginal thrush, researchers have also attempted to induce thrush in various other places on the body. The results are always consistent. You cannot take a healthy person and simply create a yeast condition without some physiological change or ill health. One type of debilitation that is sufficient for fungal invasion is an irritation or abrasion to the surface of the skin or the mucous membranes, providing that heat and moisture are also present.

Denture-wearers are more likely to find themselves with oral thrush than nondenture wearers. While there may be multiple factors involved, experts agree that the primary factor is the small areas of abrasion caused by the rubbing of the dental plates against the gums. Experiments in simulating yeast infections on the skin also show that it is not enough to apply yeast cells to the skin, then keep the area sealed off with a moist wrapping. There must be some cut or abrasion on the skin in order for an infection to become established.

Childbirth is obviously one situation where tears and abrasions can occur. Similarly, any activity that causes the genital area to become abraded, given the warmth and moisture inherent to the region, can be sufficient to trigger a yeast condition. Such situations may include times of infrequent but intense sexual relations, sex and/or masturbation with insufficient lubrication, an incorrectly fitted diaphragm, improper douching, irritation caused by excessive wiping (such as during a bladder infection), irritation from inserting tampons into a very dry vagina, and use of chemical irritants, among others.

Chemical irritation may be caused by feminine deodorant preparations (which should never be used), commercial douches, spermicides, and the contraceptive sponge. In fact, a recent study conducted in Thailand and reported in the *Journal of the American Medical Association* stated that, while the contraceptive sponge decreased the incidence of chlamydia and gonorrhea by 30 and 70 percent, respectively, it increased the incidence of yeast infections by as much as 300 percent.

Reactions to such chemicals vary among women and within your own body. Stop using any substance that causes discomfort, is highly perfumed, or is unnecessary (such as feminine deodorant preparations). Use lubricants (such as K-Y Jelly or coconut oil) before inserting anything into your vagina if you tend to be dry. By the same token, a bit of lubricant can be placed on the end of a tampon to aid insertion. Try different spermicides to find a brand and type that feels the mildest to your body. The section on "Vaginal

Care" in chapter 6 discusses these topics in more detail.

Immunosuppressant Therapy (Steroid and Cortisone Family of Drugs)

> The effect of cortisone and related substances in reducing resistance to many different types of viral, bacterial, and mycotic [fungal] infection is well recognized . . . the evidence, taken as a whole, strongly suggests that the susceptibility of the individual to Candida infections is enhanced by adrenal steroids.
>
> —Drs. Winner and Hurley, *Candida Albicans*

The healthy human body has a very high normal immunity to fungal invasion. With a limited number of exceptions, it is only in cases of extreme exposure that a healthy body will not rid itself of the invasion. This is because the healthy body has a strong immune system directing its efforts to respond appropriately to threats. When suppression of the body's natural defenses occurs, yeasts are no longer held at bay.

One of the most direct methods of suppressing the normal immunity of your body is by taking immunosuppressant medications. These include corticosteroids, anabolic steroids, and other drugs that have an immunosuppressant effect. Your immune system tries to protect your body against foreign objects (e.g., viruses, bacteria, organ transplants, etc.) by sending out an attack on the foreign substances. This is fine, unless of course, you happen to want to quell your body's natural reaction and, say, accept a transplanted organ. Similarly, there are certain conditions where you want to lessen the response of your body, something asthma and arthritis sufferers know well. Immunosuppressant drugs work by inactivating this normal immune response. The steroid family of drugs, of which cortisone is the most well-known, affords dramatic relief of pain and swelling brought about by some health maladies. Unfortunately, it is not possible to suppress just one manifestation of immunity without impairing the entire immune response. When you reduce normal immune response functions, you increase susceptibility to Candida.

Immunosuppressants are not regarded in this society with the seriousness they deserve. These are extremely powerful drugs with a myriad of potential side effects. Used for limited periods, these are true wonder drugs. They should only be taken when their use is required for medical reasons, such as bad asthma, lupus, etc. They have numerous side effects which include adrenal suppression, ulcers, osteoporosis, diabetes, muscle weakness, and skin reactions.

Some of the more common drugs used in the U.S. that have an immunosuppressant effect include:

Drug Name	Brand Name
Corticosteroids:	
Hydrocortisone	Cortef
Prednisolone	usually generic
Prednisone	Deltasone
Triamcinolone	Aristocort
Immunosuppressants:	
Imuran	Azathioprine

When immunosuppressants are used, it is advisable to pay extra attention to Candida prevention. Chapter 6 should be used as a resource for these times.

Other Weaknesses in the Immune System: Illness, Poor Nutrition, Stress

> My doctor told me that yeast infections are clearly tension-related. She says she can tell when every school in town is having finals just from the cases of yeast vaginitis that walk through the door.
>
> —College student in Florida

As we have seen, except in instances of extreme fungal exposure, it is unusual for a fungal invasion to occur when the body's normal mechanisms are functioning fully to protect it. A strong immune system is the best defense against fungal attack. Women who are HIV positive, and especially women who use drugs, have a higher susceptibility to yeast infections.

While being HIV positive results in a weakened immune system, any illness or weakness, even on a much smaller scale, means an increase in the body's susceptibility to yeast. Even if you are not sick, poor nutrition can deprive the body of the tools it needs to run optimally. Stress also increases susceptibility to diseases of all sorts, and Candida is no exception.

Poor nutrition has long been associated with fungal infections. Several culprits have been suspected although none have been proven. Zinc deficiency, even in mild cases, has been associated with recurrent vaginal candidiasis, as is iron deficiency. Deficiencies of biotin (one of the B vitamins), vitamin C, and selenium have also all been linked with the onset of vaginal infection from Candida.

Diets high in refined carbohydrates, and/or sugar (and sugar substitutes) are often cited as culprits in nutrition-related candidiasis. Sugar consumption has risen (while fiber consumption has fallen) steadily and dramatically in the Western nations, excluding periods

tions. (From 1977 to 1986, the number of American children under age ten increased nine percent, while antibiotic prescriptions for them rose 51 percent.)

Parents should be aware that antibiotic use is not always warranted. A recent study showed that 90 percent of 5,000 children recovered from ear infections uneventfully in a few days without antibiotics. Parents who find themselves feeding their children antibiotics should discuss with their health care provider concomitant antifungal therapy and/or supplementing the gastrointestinal tract with "good" bacteria to help restore a proper yeast/bacteria ratio while eradicating the disease-causing bacteria. Nystatin, a safe prescription antifungal whose taste can be masked well with grape juice, will accomplish the former while acidophilus, a type of "good" bacteria that can be purchased in health food stores, takes care of the latter.

Yeasts have been around longer than humans and will, no doubt, outlive us. Just because they are waiting in the wings for an opportunity to take over does not mean we must automatically surrender. By staying healthy and being aware of the conditions that predispose your body to yeast, you are in a position to live harmoniously with the organisms and leave their pathogenic state to someone else.

3

๛

A PRIMER ON VAGINITIS

•

> Unlike most infections and infestations, it is not
> really possible to test for the presence of Candida
> . . . This is because . . . Candida is present to some
> extent in all of us. Thus, looking for it is as pointless
> as looking for mice in a granary; they are always
> present. . . .
>
> —Leon Chaitow, *Candida Albicans*

Vaginitis is the single most common ailment triggering
phone calls and visits to the gynecologist. Every day,
every gynecologist in this country sees women concerned about vaginal infection. And of all the forms of
vaginitis, yeast vaginitis leads the pack. Yeast infections have plagued millions of women for thousands of
years—it is no surprise that myths surrounding them
continue to be spread, by uninformed health care professionals and women alike. The first section of this
chapter discusses eight of the most common myths
and separates fact from fiction.

Yeast infections, while the most common, are still
just one of the many forms of vaginitis. There are over a
dozen other conditions, which can strike concurrently

with, or independent of, Candida, but which do produce symptoms that closely resemble those of Candida. What appears to be a simple yeast infection may well be just that, but it may also be multiple infections or a nonyeast vaginitis. Through a thorough understanding of the female genital anatomy, the factors that influence it, and what signs are cause for alarm, we can make wise health care decisions. The second section of this chapter discusses the presence and diagnosis of yeast; the third examines the vaginal environment and describes some forms of vaginitis that may be mistaken for yeast infection.

The most frustrating aspect of candidiasis is not the individual infection, but the repeat nature of the illness. When coupled with other medical maladies, the situation can be overwhelming. If you suffer from health conditions that have evaded successful diagnosis or treatment (irritable colon, skin problems, or constipation, for example), there is a possibility that the yeast in your body is playing a pivotal role in your current state of health. The final section of this chapter discusses the possibility that other medical conditions may be associated with yeast overgrowth and/or a yeast hypersensitivity, and suggests some strategies for testing and treating this.

The Myths of Yeast Infections

MYTH 1:
Use of the Pill is not related to your chronic yeast infections

The Pill is, overwhelmingly, the most popular form of birth control in America today. There are many wonderful things about the Pill. For both doctor and patient, it is the simplest form of birth control available. One prescription is all it takes—no messy exam or lengthy office visit, no spermicides or applicators, no interruption of sexual excitement to insert a barrier— and best of all, it has the highest degree of reliability of all the currently available methods of birth control.

Unfortunately, over 25 years of research has consistently found that women who use oral contraceptives are significantly more likely to suffer from vaginal candidiasis. Studies, as early as 1964, began reporting that women on the Pill were far more likely to find themselves with a yeast infection, and a further two decades of research has confirmed the results, even with the lower dosage pills now available.

To make matters worse, the effects of the Pill increase over time. The longer you stay on the Pill, the more likely you are to find yourself with an infection. In a major piece of research examining more than 8,000 women over six years, there was a significantly higher incidence of yeast vaginitis only in patients who had taken the Pill for more than 12 months. Similarly, a 1971 study found that women taking the Pill usually required double or triple the normal dose of antifungal therapy in order to clear the yeast vaginitis; in some cases, it was necessary to discontinue the Pill before a cure could be achieved at all.

These results should not be the least bit surprising if you remember that the Pill works, roughly, by tricking your body into thinking it is pregnant by inducing hormonal changes which correspond closely to those of pregnancy. Pregnancy is known to be a significant precursor to yeast infections with pregnant women reporting yeast vaginitis twenty times more frequently than nonpregnant women. Specifically, the Pill produces changes in both the content and pH of the vagina, changes which, in turn, alter the vaginal environment so that it becomes quite favorable to Candida.

Though this connection between birth control hormones and yeast vaginitis should not be the least bit shocking, some doctors do not acknowledge the possibility. They insist that the Pill is not only safe and effective, but that it has no side effects whatsoever. When questioned by patients about their chronic recurrences of candidiasis, these M.D.s simply shrug their shoulders.

Any women suffering from recurrent yeast vaginitis should know that the Pill is more than likely contributing to the problem. Switching from the Pill to a barrier method of birth control lowers your likelihood of infection by all microorganisms, providing you with not only a lowered yeast susceptibility, but with a higher resistance to vaginal infections of all kinds.

MYTH 2:
You can't catch it from, or give it to, a sexual partner

Transmission of the yeast organism between humans has been noted in the medical literature since the last century. Candida can be propagated by direct contact as well as by inadvertent indirect contact with sites of yeast colonization. A baby's oral thrush from a mother's infected nipple and diaper rash (thrush) from contact with the infected hands of a caretaker are both examples. Genital transmission provides another route of contracting Candida. In fact, for record-keeping purposes, the Centers for Disease Control in Atlanta classifies candidiasis as a sexually transmitted disease.

When my husband and I were still dating, he was living in New York and I was here. We'd see each other about every month and a half. I'd get a yeast infection by the Monday of each weekend we were together. I'd never had them ever before. When I asked my doctor about it, he said that the yeast was a problem within my body and that the timing with my boyfriend's visits was merely coincidental.

—Maria, 31-year-old chef in Atlanta

One 1977 article reported that yeasts were probably spread by sexual transmission in 30–40 percent of the cases of genital candidiasis studied. Another article found that 15 percent of yeast vaginitis patients provided a positive history connecting sexual intercourse to symptomatic Candida infections. Two yeast researchers in 1973 concluded that because the organism may be transmitted sexually, it is usually wise to treat sex partners lest treated women quickly become reinfected.

Yet despite the evidence that women can infect, and be infected from, a sexual partner, many doctors do not acknowledge this possibility. They insist that yeast infections bear no relationship to sexual activity and that any link between the two is likely to be due more to a woman's emotional health than to any contribution from the partner. (Some doctors, while insisting that it is essentially impossible for a circumcised male to infect a woman through sex, will acquiesce that an uncircumcised male can pass the yeast organisms.)

When there is even a suspected link between yeast infections and sexual activity, leaving the partner untreated sets the woman up for continuing infections and reduces the likelihood that her treatment will be successful. Reducing the yeast in the partner may or may not be the sole solution to the cycle of infection, but, at the very least, it will eliminate one mode for reinfection and thus should be an integral part of the treatment program.

So if you sense a link between sexual activity and subsequent symptoms of an infection or if you have a regular partner, male or female, and can't seem to eliminate repeat infections, you definitely should explore treating your partner(s). (See chapter 5 for treatment information.)

MYTH 3:
If you just wait, your menstrual cycle will "cleanse out" the infection

For many women, the onset of menses is an emotional marker. It is a reminder that another cycle has passed, an indicator that the "plumbing" is all in working order (unless you are trying to become pregnant, in which case, it is a profoundly depressing experience). Finally, it provides an internal calendar by which the events in life can be measured. For some, it is also viewed as a time of refreshing and renewing the body, menses being the body's way of cleansing out impurities so that the cycle can start each month fresh and clean. But this notion of the flowing blood cleansing out the body could not be more incorrect for women who are susceptible to yeast infections.

> I used to get so distraught. I would get infections a lot right before my period. I thought it was great timing because I figured my period would literally wash the infection away. When my period was over, the infection would always be there. I had no idea that "that time of the month" was when I was most likely to get them, and that the timing was no coincidence.
>
> —Sandy, a 29-year-old from Washington, D.C.

The days immediately before and during your period are prime time for yeast infection. This is so for several reasons. First, you may experience premenstrual symptoms, such as a sweet tooth or cramps, which may lower your nutritional state and increase your level of stress and fatigue. Sugar is the last thing you should consume when you are susceptible because it actually feeds the yeast. Also, any time your overall health is diminished (as with PMS), you become susceptible to infections of all sorts.

Second, your vaginal pH maintains itself at a fairly constant level through the monthly cycle, varying narrowly between 3.8 and 4.5. As we know, larger fluctuations in pH alter the chemical environment making it increasingly favorable for certain organisms (such as *Candida albicans*) to flourish while others (such as some of the yeast-fighting bacteria) die off. As you approach menstruation, the pH rises, reaching its highest point during your menstrual flow. At this time, it may be as high as 6.8, due both to hormonal activity and the fact that blood has a higher alkalinity than the normal vaginal fluids. These fluctuations in the pH mean that a normally stable environment is not so stable one week out of each month.

Third, the menstrual blood itself is a highly nutritious food supply for yeast. The combination of the blood's warmth, moisture, and nutrient content has a growth-enhancing effect on the yeast. Combine a lower resistance, altered pH, and warm food source for the yeast, and you have a perfect recipe for growing yeast once a month.

Since the days surrounding your period are your most susceptible, that is when the most effort should be directed at minimizing the possibility of an infection. It is possible to manage the environment, but you can't do this if you don't know what factors make a difference. Chapter 6 has information that will help you stop the yeast before it can get started.

MYTH 4:

Women with any type of vaginal problem should never wear tampons

It is a common belief that, if something is wrong in the vaginal region, the last thing you should do is stick something "up there." Toxic Shock Syndrome (TSS) also helped give tampons a bad name. However, women battling with the pain and discharge of yeast infections do not have to endure the mess and inconvenience of wearing pads as well. A 1984 study found that women who rely on tampons (rather than napkins or pads) during menstruation have candidiasis *significantly less* frequently than women using sanitary napkins only. There may be several reasons for this. First, napkins become damp and stay damp, providing yeasts with the moisture they need to survive. Second, pads close off the vaginal opening, creating a warm, moist, self-contained ecosystem for yeast growth. Finally, the anus is harboring its own population of yeast. Pads may act as an infection link between the anus and the vagina.

Whether to use tampons or pads during an infection is a question of personal preference. If you prefer to use pads, be sure to change them frequently and try to wash and dry your external genitalia several times a day with a mild soap. If you prefer tampons, avoid the superabsorbent varieties (these are the ones associated with TSS), scented or deodorant tampons (the chemicals may be irritating), or any brand that causes discomfort during insertion or wear. In general, the use of tampons during a yeast infection is not only allowable, but seems preferred.

MYTH 5:
Yeast infections will go away by themselves if just ignored

The first couple of times I got an infection I just didn't have the money to go to the doctor. I decided to try to live with the itching. By my next cycle it had got so much worse, I just couldn't stand it. Finally, I went to the doctor and got some Monistat. It provided immediate relief, but the infection always came back with my period after that.

—Tina, a graduate student in Denver

When you have to decide whether or not to respond to a new infection, it is always easier and cheaper to do nothing and hope that it will go away by itself. A yeast infection may, in fact, go away untreated. For example, if you get them only occasionally there is a chance that, left alone, the vaginal environment will return to normal, the yeast will subside, and the infection will vanish. However, once yeasts get a foothold, they are very reluctant to relinquish control. The infection which goes away on its own is, unfortunately, the exception rather than the rule.

Because the yeast is growing *in response* to some other condition, it and the infection it causes are unlikely to go away unless you address whatever factors predisposed you to it in the first place. When such infections do clear up spontaneously, there is a significant likelihood of a return within a month or two. Recurrence is the hallmark of this disease. Yeast is your body telling you that something is out of kilter. This is the perfect time to analyze why you might have become susceptible to yeast, and how you can best rebuild your natural resistance. Chances are that if you ignore the yeast indicator now, it will simply get worse until you can't ignore it any longer.

MYTH 6:
Yeast infections are simply a normal part of being female

> The most infuriating part of having the infections all the time was that my doctor said it was normal. Here I was, my discharge smelly and my crotch in so much pain I can barely pee, and he's telling me it's normal. It was about as normal as an infant having a migraine headache!
>
> —Christa, a marketing analyst in Houston

In some cases, when prescription antifungals are unable to cure a condition, it is frequently attributed to psychosomatic causes or written off altogether as being "normal." Often, too, when a condition is widespread, the label "common" gets distorted and becomes interpreted as "normal." Women with recurrent yeast vaginitis have been diagnosed as being psychologically unstable and even chastised for complaining about something that isn't a "real" problem. As callous and disturbing as this is, it implies even more horribly the lack of concern needed to push the effort to prevent or cure yeast infections.

For years, severe premenstrual syndrome was seen as an emotional problem, a sign of an unstable personality. Now we know that women with severe PMS should be tested and treated for certain nutritional imbalances and, possibly, endometriosis. Obese people, for example, today have tests for thyroid problems that may cause their obesity rather than being dismissed by doctors simply as "severely lacking in willpower."

Yeast infections are just one of many illnesses whose presence has been called "normal" simply because its manifestation and treatment are not well understood by the medical community. The word *disease* literally means "lacking ease." If you have chronic yeast vaginitis, you are more than likely dis-eased, and no explanation that the condition is "normal" should ever suffice. If your current doctor is unwilling to work with you in resolving the problem, find a health practitioner who is.

MYTH 7:
All women with recurring vaginitis should be tested for diabetes

Almost every treatise on yeast infections emphasizes the need to exclude latent diabetes as a possible explanation of frequent recurrences. It is assumed that, in many cases, recurring yeast problems are an indicator of the onset of diabetes.

The candidiasis/diabetes link is based on the fact that diabetics maintain higher levels of sugar in their bodies, and sugar can act as a food source for yeasts. Sugar-laden urine around the vaginal opening is presumed to be a suitable culture medium for vaginal yeast; as well, the higher levels of sugar in the bloodstream of a diabetic are thought to increase susceptibility.

The suspicion of diabetes can be easily eliminated by undergoing a simple glucose tolerance test. While a precautionary diabetes test is not difficult, almost no women with recurrent infections are found to have any indicators at all of the disease. In fact, the diabetes/candidiasis link is assumed more from repetition than from reality, something evident in its citation as a condition to test for in almost every medical text on the subject.

Although the glucose tolerance test for diabetes has been performed on thousands of women with yeast infections, the percentage who turn out to be even slightly diabetic is close to zero. The 1984 International Symposium on Vulvovaginal Mycoses concluded: *Since the pickup rate of diabetes is almost nil, the test is a waste of time.* Similarly, a study reported the same year found that *in hundreds of patients with recurrent vulvovaginal candidiasis, laboratory testing failed to identify a single diabetic.*

Performing the test is not only more wasted time and money, it also causes unnecessary emotional stress while you wait to learn the results. Worrying about how you are going to manage diabetes when you can't even manage your vaginitis can be frightening. Also, ironically, if the doctor has lead you to believe that diabetes is the probable culprit, it can be disappointing to get a negative result for it suggests, even more than before, that your illness is a real freak of nature.

The last word: If your family has a strong history of diabetes; you are obese; loosing weight despite eating and urinating frequently; are postmenopausal, or breast-feeding, you should be screened for diabetes. Your preadolescent children should be tested if they suffer persistently or repeatedly from such infections. Buy an inexpensive finger-stick glucose test can (sold at drugstores) and do the test at home if you do want to check yourself first for diabetes.

MYTH 8:
Intermittent prophylactic therapy is the best treatment approach

For many doctors frustrated with their patients who have recurrent infections, Intermittent Prophylactic Therapy (IPT) has become the default remedy. This generally means the patient uses a nystatin or imidazole suppository or cream (such as Monistat) once or twice a day every month around the time of menstruation.

IPT is unfortunately only a stopgap measure that burdens you with the cost of expensive medications for only temporary relief. Such treatment is expensive, messy, and inconvenient, and it merely skirts around the facts—that an illness is present and recurring. If a yeast infection is your body's way of telling you that there is a problem, IPT is the equivalent of wearing earplugs.

The problem is that IPT is simply not effective with no evidence that it decreases the likelihood of repeat infections. Clinical studies have found that IPT kept symptoms below a critical level but did not affect the return of yeasts to the vagina. Rather than an effective treatment, IPT tends to mask the condition. As most IPT prescriptions are for multiple refills, you can treat yourself for a long time independently when a different treatment strategy or a reevaluation of the diagnosis may be more appropriate. While antifungal medications can provide short-term relief, allowing a breather from the pain, you should focus instead on beginning a complete treatment program that addresses underlying causes and predisposing factors.

When Is Yeast Responsible for the Infection

The isolation of fungi is a relatively easy procedure; the identification and determination of significance is much more difficult.

—John Rippon, *Medical Mycology*

If you suspect you have a yeast infection and seek medical attention, you can expect to receive a pelvic exam, which normally includes a culture or microscopic analysis of your vaginal secretions. Very often, the technician or lab will report that Candida is present in your secretions. There are three criteria that the practitioner may then use in determining the significance of this finding: the mere presence of yeast, the biological stage of the yeast, and the quantity of yeast. These approaches to diagnosis may be interesting intellectually, but, as we will see, are of very little clinical significance. Let's look at them one at a time.

Is the mere presence of yeast in the vagina enough to satisfy a diagnosis of a yeast infection? There are a number of opinions on this topic. Since yeasts often, but not always, appear in a microscopic examination of vaginal discharge (of both infected and noninfected women), we must start by asking whether or not the presence in itself is meaningful. Medically put, when is it that the discovery of Candida should or should not be regarded as pathological?

At one time, doctors felt that *C. albicans* was not part of the normal vaginal flora, suspecting that its presence was an indicator of disease. That opinion is no longer held by most researchers. While some doctors believe that *Candida albicans* was not part of the resident flora of the vagina, many others believe that there may be a state of happy symbiosis in which the fungus lives in the vagina but causes no harm until one of the predisposing factors becomes operative. Some have attempted to use the different spellings to distinguish the two situations: candidosis being the condition where candida organisms in the vagina are causing irritation, candidiasis being the condition where candida organisms in the vagina are residing harmlessly. This term distinction, however, never took hold.

A 1975 British study found that more than half of the women seen who were harboring *C. albicans* were not complaining and had no obvious clinical manifestations of infection. Another study published in 1977 determined that women with or without symptoms could have the same yeast count. Additional studies have demonstrated that the presence of asymptomatic vaginal colonization with Candida occurs in approximately 10 to 55 percent of healthy adult women. Most investigators, however, estimate the incidence at closer to 15 to 20 percent.

As many as one-quarter of all healthy women may then test positively for vaginal Candida with absolutely no signs whatsoever of infection. These findings have led most health practitioners to acknowledge that simply finding the organism in the vagina is not an indication for treatment. Management of this disease rests not with eradication of all bodily yeasts but with long-term relief of symptoms.

A second approach researchers have taken in trying to determine when yeast is pathological is to examine the biological form of the yeast organism when it is found in the vagina or rectum. Yeast can be observed in what is termed the "yeast stage" or the "sprouting mycelial form." It has been postulated that the former is a harmless, noninvasive, sugar-fermenting organism, while the latter produces rhizoids, or very long root structures, which can penetrate the mucosa and become invasive.

Many workers have found the pathogenicity of *C. albicans* to vary with its [form] . . . Most of these reports suggest that the mycelial phase is invasive, but that the yeast-cell phase is not. . . . There appears no clear-cut distinction in pathogenicity between the mycelial and the yeast phases of *C. albicans.*

> —Drs. Winner and Hurley, *Candida Albicans*

Although the issue has been studied for well over 20 years, it continues to surface in literature and practice. Some practitioners use yeast form as a clear diagnostic tool: They examine a specimen under the microscope, and if mycelial growths are seen, they take it as fact that disease is present. As the number of women with yeast-related illnesses has increased, this unsubstantiated yeast form distinction is appearing increasingly in the literature.

> There has appeared a surfeit of literature concerning the relative pathogenicity of the mycelial and the yeast stage of *Candida albicans.* It was felt that the sprouting of the yeast cell to form mycelium . . . was necessary for invasion of tissue. . . . The inflammatory, toxic, and invasive abilities of *C. albicans* are a *characteristic of the species* and not of a particular growth form. (Emphasis added by authors)

> —John Rippon, *Medical Mycology*

A practitioner who seeks to diagnose and treat you on the basis of yeast form may sound convincing, but such a diagnosis is founded on myth.

A third technique used to determine if the Candida found in the vaginal secretions is pathological or not is by measuring the quantity of yeast organisms present (called "yeast load") and to declare illness based on a numeric measure of Candida organisms.

Quantities of yeast organisms can provide some good insight into the severity of the problem. In many women, there is a correlation between amount of yeast and amount of illness. While there is not an absolute correlation between symptoms and yeast load, the majority of symptomatic women do have large numbers of yeast present in their vaginal secretions.

However, a direct relationship between quantity of yeast and symptoms is not always the case, nor should it be assumed. There is little evidence that patients with vaginal candidiasis yield higher concentrations of Candida than those without clinical disease.

While finding out how many thousands of yeast organisms are present in your discharge may be fascinating, it is not revealing in and of itself. Unless you know what your normal colonization rate is (which is difficult, as the number varies), a colonization rate measured while an infection is present provides you with a number, but no context—making it more interesting than useful.

If we cannot determine disease by the presence, form, or concentration of yeast, where does that leave us in discovering when the discharge or discomfort is due to Candida?

The answer is actually quite simple. *Yeast should be considered pathological when there are clear clinical symptoms or signs of Candida and negative findings for any other pathogen.* Simply put, the mere presence of yeast is not the issue; the symptoms of yeast, absent any other disease-producing entities, make it an issue.

The following sections review the vaginal environment and the symptoms of yeast and non-yeast infections alike to ensure you have all the information you need for good vaginal health.

Vaginitis

This section is broken into three parts. The first part examines a healthy vaginal environment and explains some of the mechanisms at play. The second part details the symptoms of yeast vaginitis; the third describes other forms of vaginitis that produce symptoms which can imitate those of yeast vaginitis.

The general term for any of the many reproductive tract problems involving irritation or inflammation of the vagina is *vaginitis*. Before we look more in depth at yeast and non-yeast vaginitis, we'll take a look at what is happening in a healthy vaginal environment in order to understand when and how deviations from normal occur.

What constitutes a "normal" vaginal environment varies from one woman to another. A healthy vagina can harbor up to 29 different species of organisms, but there is no exact combination of genital microflora normal for all females. The flora will differ depending on such factors as age, hormone levels, menses and type of menstrual protection, degree and diversity of sexual activity, type of contraceptive method, drug use (especially antibiotics), and any history of genital surgical procedures. The type and amount of vaginal discharge varies not only from woman to woman, but also in each part of every woman's menstrual cycle. The same holds true for vaginal odors. Like snowflakes, no two women are necessarily identical, nor are you, microbiologically speaking, the same as you were a week ago.

The healthy vagina is a self-maintaining ecosystem that needs no intervention. It cleanses itself daily. It is kept moist by slight discharge from the cervix and vaginal walls. The fact that the normal discharge flows downward allows old cells, menstrual blood, and other matter to be routinely carried out of the vagina. There are no glands in the vagina; the fluid it contains results from cervical secretion and from "sweating" (called transudation) through the vaginal wall. Normal vaginal discharge contains: clear watery mucus from the cervix (especially around ovulation); clear fluid that has transuded through the walls of the vagina (especially during sexual excitement, but also during pregnancy or emotional upset); dead cells from the vaginal walls; and fluid excreted during sexual excitement from the Bartholin's glands (at the vaginal entrance). The resulting discharge is transparent or slightly milky, with little or no odor, slippery in feel, and sometimes yellowish when it dries.

Certain changes in the vagina occur naturally and are somewhat predictable. For instance, a change in the quantity and quality of discharge occurs with the monthly cycle, being most noticeable immediately before and during ovulation. At this time, your mucous becomes thicker and slicker (with an ability to stretch) in order to help the sperm reach the cervical opening on its journey toward fertilization. This change in discharge should not be a cause for concern. Changes in the type or amount of discharge at other times, however, may warrant further investigation. Since we cannot point to an objective definition for normal, your familiarity with your own body will ultimately be your main diagnostic tool.

The key to determining if there is some condition that needs attention is whether there is anything unusual from within or around the vagina. Any noticeable increase or change in amount or quality of vaginal discharge, especially if accompanied by odor, tenderness, or pain, is an indication that you may have vaginitis.

The chief symptoms of vaginitis are sudden, abnormal discharge, generally followed by itching and soreness of the vagina and external genitalia. Usually it is an infection brought on by a fungus, bacterium, or other microscopic parasite and can stem from one or multiple sources. Chemicals in commercial douches, vaginal sprays, even super-absorbent tampons can cause irritation or infection. Vaginitis can result from bacteria from the feces getting into the vagina. Irritations from insufficient lubrication during sexual intercourse can also produce vaginitis.

Vaginitis can be "caught" from a partner, who may or may not have symptoms. Sometimes infections are not the result of invasion by an outside organism (such as trichomonas), but from an overgrowth of organisms which normally live harmlessly within the body (such as Candida). This overgrowth may be due to an altering of the pH or chemical balance of the vagina. Excessive douching, antibiotics, oral contraceptives, pregnancy, and diabetes are some of the factors that can alter the chemical makeup. As with all infections, vaginitis is more likely to take hold when your resistance is lowered—by poor diet, stress, or illness (including PMS).

If you notice an increase in the quantity or a change in the quality of your discharge, be sure to check that you haven't left a tampon, contraceptive or menstrual sponge, or cervical cap or diaphragm in your vagina. These can cause a very thick, odorous discharge, which will clear up as soon as the object is removed.

Some women interested in measuring their fertility levels, either to achieve or avoid pregnancy, track their vaginal mucus. While this is normally a good indicator, it may not be reliable if you have vaginitis because you probably won't be able to tell the difference between normal mucus and the discharge resulting from an infection or particular medication. You should not rely on mucus observation for birth control if you suspect you have vaginitis. Also, be careful not to confuse mucus with semen or secretions during sexual arousal;

while spermicidal foams, creams, and jellies are in your vagina, you probably won't be able to distinguish cervical from other discharge.

Of all the forms of vaginitis, yeast infections (caused by *Candida albicans*) are the most common. *Trichomonas* and *gardnerella* round out the list for the most common types of vaginitis.

Diagnosing your own infections without a doctor is relatively easy, especially once you've had a few.

> I can tell I have an infection coming on a few days before there are any signs. There's a certain tingling and it stings just a little when I urinate. Sure enough, the discharge starts soon and it gets a bit puffy "down there." There's also the smell, kind of a nice smell actually, like a bakery really early in the morning.
>
> —Sasha, 41-year-old cashier

The telltale signs of a candida infection are a thick white discharge that looks like cottage cheese and smells like baking bread. The external genitalia become red and swollen, often with intense itching, and there may be pain during urination and intercourse. Some women also experience an outbreak similar to diaper rash in the skin surrounding the vagina and anus. While you may have all these classic symptoms and signs, you might find yourself with just one or two of these along with, potentially, a few symptoms unique to you.

Candida is, of course, not the only organism that can result in symptoms such as discharge and odor. It is possible to have multiple infections, in which case treating the yeast alone may not be sufficient. Once the yeast has established a real foothold, you may need treatment for all the infections. However, Candida may be just the secondary infection, taking advantage of the compromised environment; in which case, treating the primary infection may be sufficient to make the region inhospitable to yeast.

The most common infection mix is trichomonas with gardnerella. Studies have reported up to 35 percent of patients with trichomonas testing positive for gardnerella as well. Conversely, gardnerella and yeast are almost mutually exclusive—the environment that supports one cannot support the other.

The most important thing in treating any problem is knowing exactly what the cause is. In the case of yeast, clinical self-diagnosis will most likely tell you as much as any medical test. (Chapter 4 lists the situations in which you should seek a medical opinion even if you are fairly certain yeast is the culprit.) With all other reproductive tract infections, however, self-diagnosis can be much more difficult, if not impossible. If there is any question in your mind about the nature of your infection, have a health care practitioner perform a complete pelvic exam.

The main reason to see a professional is not to see if you have yeast—it is to make sure you don't have anything else. Yeast infections, fortunately, will not cause lasting physical damage; they do not harm the uterus or tubes and will not threaten fertility. Unfortunately, this is not true for many of the other forms of vaginitis. If vaginitis is present, yet you feel confident that it is a yeast infection just like the ones you've had before and nothing in your life has changed much, and you are not pregnant, there may be no reason to look further than your medicine chest and drug or health food store. But, you must seek medical consultation if:

• you have had only a few yeast infections and are really not sure whether the current infection is the same type as the earlier ones;

- you have a new sexual partner, you have multiple partners, or your sexual partner(s) have new partners;
- you have any symptom of anything other than those associated with a classic yeast infection (see page 1);
- you feel you have a classic yeast infection, but the treatments that have always worked before aren't working;
- you are confident that you have a yeast infection, but prefer to use prescription treatments and cannot get a prescription without seeing a medical doctor;
- you've recently gone through a physiological change, i.e., puberty, pregnancy, menopause.

Having a general knowledge of the organisms and conditions that can affect the reproductive region will help you identify the symptoms you have and thus make the appropriate response. Yeast will respond well to home remedies, and some pathogens can be left alone. Other pathogens, however, require immediate medical attention.

Listed below are the names and descriptions of additional reproductive tract diseases that could possibly be mistaken for yeast. Remember, the symptoms of yeast vaginitis include vaginal itching; a white discharge resembling cottage cheese and sometimes with a yeasty smell like that of baking bread; a reddened, swollen vaginal area; and a burning sensation, especially when urinating or having intercourse.

The listing does not include every potential vaginal disease (for instance, syphilis and lice), but does cover all the major culprits producing unusual discharge—the primary problem indicator.

Trichomonas Vaginitis, or "trich," is caused by

trichomonas, a microscopic one-celled parasite. It can cause disease in both men and women, occurring alone or with gonorrhea and chlamydia. The organisms can be easily identified by examination of a wet smear or by culture of the vaginal discharge. The organisms cause small, deep red spots to appear on the cervix. Trichomonas infections do not cause damage to the body and need not be treated.

Trich affects 2.5 million American women each year. Symptoms of trich infection are severe itching and a frothy, bubbly, profuse vaginal discharge, yellowish green or gray in color with a distinctive foul (sometimes "fishy") odor. Urination and intercourse may be painful, and women with trich have twice the rate of endometritis. If the infection spreads into the bladder area, it can cause a urinary tract infection, with a primary symptom being the desire to urinate all the time even though the bladder is empty. A lab test may return positive for trich after a routine pelvic exam, but again, if no symptoms are apparent, treatment is not required.

Trichomonas is without question sexually transmitted. It has its highest incidence among those in their sexually active years and among those most sexually active. In trials using healthy female volunteers, researchers have found it very difficult to establish an infection even when these women were inoculated with large numbers of trichomonads; in fact, it is almost never seen in adult virgins. It is almost always contracted through intercourse. There is a high degree of sexual transmission: female sexual partners of infected men are almost certain to get it, male partners of infected women get trich 60–76 percent of the time. Trich organisms do not survive in the mouth, thus oral sex is not implicated in its transmission. The trich organisms can survive in moist places for several hours, so take care to wipe your vagina from front to back, use clean towels and washcloths, sterile douche tips, and dry toilet seats.

Emotional stress can cause symptoms to flare up or recur. It tends to occur more frequently in the winter. And because the trich organisms flourish best in an alkaline environment, women are more susceptible to it during and after menstruation. Reinfection can be a problem for some women.

Home remedies include vinegar douches to help acidify the vagina. *The Medical SelfCare Book of Women's Health* describes a specific douche recipe for trich: combine four tablespoons plain white vinegar with one or two drops of baby shampoo in a quart of warm water. Douche with the mixture daily for one week, then twice weekly for a month or more. The trichomonas organism is damaged by the acidity of the vinegar and its cell wall may be destroyed by the detergent in the baby shampoo. [For more information on douching, see chapter 5.] Natamycin, a topical antifungal, is successful in treating trich.

For severe or recurrent cases of trich, the standard treatment is with oral and intravaginal metronidazole (Flagyl). All sexual partners should be treated simultaneously, even though all may not be symptomatic. The cure rate for women increases when sexual partners are treated simultaneously. You should also use condoms during intercourse while undergoing treatment. Flagyl may be taken in one large single dose, a slightly smaller double dose, or in much smaller doses three times a day over a one-week period. Flagyl can cause serious side effects and therefore should not be used by women who are pregnant or nursing, or by those with peptic ulcers or central nervous system disorders. Side effects may include nausea, headache, diarrhea, dry mouth, convulsive seizures, and numbness in the limbs. Abstain from all alcoholic beverages during treatment and for two days after.

Gardnerella Vaginitis, also known as Hemophilus, was first described in 1955. It is a bacterial infection that thrives when the normal pH of the vagina is raised to alkaline levels. It can be transmitted through sexual intercourse, from douche nozzles, toilet seats, washcloths and towels, or arise spontaneously. The symptoms are similar to those of trich, with the discharge a homogeneous creamy white or grayish, and an especially foul smell, like "rotten fish" after intercourse.

The gardnerella organism does not affect the vaginal tissues, so signs of irritation such as itching, burning, and soreness are characteristically absent. Because this form of vaginitis does not cause inflammation, nearly 75 percent of women with gardnerella have no symptoms in the early stages. Characteristic symptoms are discharge and odor. Since it is not a tissue pathogen, there is little need to treat it unless the symptoms are sufficiently bothersome. As with Candida, it is the patient's complaints that matter, not simply the presence of the gardnerella organism.

Clinicians diagnose gardnerella by the presence of "clue cells," identified microscopically from vaginal discharge, but don't be surprised if your doctor also finds *Candida albicans*. Studies show that either the Candida or the gardnerella may be present without causing discomfort because the microbiologic environment necessary to sustain one as a vaginal pathogen effectively precludes *functional* significance of the other. In other words, if your doctor informs you that both organisms are present, you should know that, first, neither has to be treated unless you are experiencing pain or discomfort and that, second, only one is causing the problem. A review of symptoms should reveal which one.

Like trich, gardnerella will not threaten a woman's fertility and simultaneous treatment of partners is recommended (which is a bit ironic since there has never been a drug approved for treating men). During a gardnerella infection, the pH has generally risen, so increasing the acidity of the vagina is in order. The most common home remedy is a povidone-iodine douche (see pages 188–90) which can be purchased over-the-counter in most drugstores (but should not be used by pregnant women). Flagyl (see trich, above), oral ampicillin, or an antibiotic cream containing sulfa (e.g., Triple Sultrin) are the common prescription remedies. Be aware that sulfa allergy and sensitivity is not uncommon. If you or your partners are allergic to penicillin, do not take ampicillin. If you do take ampicillin or any antibiotic, be sure to use an antifungal regime to counter the effects of the drug to ward off a yeast infection (see the "Guide to Taking Antibiotics" in chapter 6).

Chlamydia annually affects millions of men and women, primarily between the ages of twenty to twenty-four. Chlamydia can lead to severe pelvic inflammatory disease (PID), sterility, infection of the urethra and cervix, and complications in babies born to infected mothers. It is caused by bacteria that are spread through vaginal or anal sex with an infected partner, but it can also be passed by hand from the discharge of an infected eye.

Unfortunately, chlamydia symptoms may go unnoticed often and, only one partner will have them though the other can be an asymptomatic carrier. Symptoms may include yellowish discharge, reddened, tender cervix, pain during intercourse or urination, and unusual bleeding. In men, symptoms may include thin, watery penile discharge along with burning around the urethra and during urination.

Chlamydia is often found in people with gonorrhea symptoms, but with negative gonococcal cultures. It can be diagnosed by culture or by a direct antibody test (called Microtrak). Since the antibody test can give false negatives, it is safest to have both tests performed.

All partners must undergo treatment since reinfection from an asymptomatic partner is possible. Antibiotics, most commonly a tetracycline taken four times a day, are effective against the chlamydia bacterium. It is best to avoid intimate contact until you are certain that you and your partner(s) are cured. If you do need to take antibiotics, be sure to get an antifungal to counter the likelihood of developing a yeast infection (see the "Guide to Taking Antibiotics" in chapter 6).

Gonorrhea is not new and thus receives little media attention, but it remains a highly contagious sexually transmitted disease with serious implications. The good news is that it is fully curable, the bad news that, if undetected, it can lead to sterility, blindness, and death. Known as the clap, drip, dose, strain, or GC, it is caused by a bacterium and is spread through sexual intercourse, genital-oral, and genital-rectal sex.

Symptoms usually occur within two to twenty days after exposure. Sadly, over half of the women infected with gonorrhea remain asymptomatic or have symptoms mild enough to be ignored or confused with other problems, a real danger. The first clue may be an itchy discharge or burning on you or your partner. If symptoms do occur, they may include redness and small bumps on the cervix, unusual discharge, pain during urination or intercourse, pelvic tenderness, vaginal bleeding, or fever. Many cases, though, are only detected by a routine gonorrhea culture performed during a gynecological exam.

It is crucial to take active measures against this disease since its effects can be devastating, including joint pain, sterility, and blindness. Additionally, gonorrhea is more likely to persist and spread in women than in men. As *My Body, My Health: The Concerned Women's Guide to Gynecology* explains, a man who has intercourse once with an infected woman has a 20–25 percent chance of becoming infected, but a woman who has intercourse just once with an infected man is almost certain to become infected. It may easily spread to your tubes and uterus if you have intercourse during your period, because the bacteria thrive on blood.

Statistically, most cases of gonorrhea in women occur during the late teen years and in the early twenties. Cases of gonorrhea in women over 30 make up a minuscule percentage of the total number of cases. A culture must be taken to accurately determine the presence of the gonococcal organisms. Cervical sampling is best, but throat and anal cultures should also be taken if you have had oral-genital contact or anal intercourse. The culture tests will take about 48 hours. A blood test for syphilis should be taken as well since it is not unusual for the two infections to coexist.

Treatment with antibiotics can completely eradicate the disease. Remember that antibiotics must be taken in the correct dosage and for the prescribed duration to be effective. Again, all partners will need to be treated with antibiotics as well. It is best to avoid all intercourse and oral sex until you are certain that you and your partner(s) are cured. If you do need to take antibiotics, be sure to get an antifungal to counter a yeast infection.

Contracting gonorrhea during pregnancy poses very serious risks. Prompt treatment is essential.

Herpes is a viral infection whose incidence has skyrocketed in the last decade. Though not normally considered a vaginitis, herpes causes itching as a major symptom and this can be confused with yeast vaginitis, especially in the early stages. The telltale sign of herpes is blisters or fever sores, found either in and around the mouth (Type 1 Herpes) and/or in and around the genital region (Type 2 Herpes). Intercourse is not required to transmit the disease. Simple skin contact with the open sores is sufficient. Herpes can be passed from mouth to mouth, mouth to genitals (and vice versa), and genitals to genitals.

Once infected, the herpes virus lives in the body permanently, feeding off the nutrients in the cells. As with all viruses, there is no cure. The virus may stay dormant or may become active at any time.

Symptoms appear from two days to four weeks after exposure (three days is average). An outbreak usually begins with a tingling, burning, or itching sensation of the skin in the genital area, sometimes with a minor rash. Small painful blisters that rupture with a watery discharge, and then heal are the telltale sign. Urination may be painful and there might be a sharp burning pain in the entire genital area. Abnormal discharge often accompanies the blisters. Sometimes though, the only symptoms may be swelling and reddening of the genital area, itching, or discharge. When no open sores appear, herpes is more likely to be misdiagnosed. Generally the first outbreak is the most painful and takes the longest to heal.

Herpes is contagious when your sores are open, but it is difficult to say how long it remains contagious once the sores begin to heal. No one knows at what exact stage in the healing process the risk of infecting a partner is over. Intercourse, as well as oral sex, should be avoided until the sores are completely healed. If you choose to engage in intercourse before the sores are totally healed, use a condom. Once the sores are completely healed, no precautions need to be taken.

The virus is particularly reactive to stress with many people reporting that stress, more than diet, exercise, or pharmaceutical use, is the primary determinant of secondary outbreaks.

Herpes sores will heal and disappear by themselves, but recurrent episodes are likely. Some lucky individuals will suffer flare-ups only occasionally, but five to eight outbreaks a year is the norm. When sores are active, herpes can usually be recognized by sight, but misdiagnosis does occur. A laboratory exam can confirm the diagnosis.

All of the treatments for herpes are aimed at reducing the frequency, severity, and duration of the outbreaks, since there is no known cure. The amino acid, L-Lysine (available at health food stores) is the most popular self-help treatment. A dosage of 750–1,000 milligrams per day (taken with meals) when symptoms appear and 500 milligrams per day at other times is recommended. Daily doses of zinc are also said to be helpful, 25 milligrams daily for maintenance, 50 milligrams daily during symptoms. Povidone-iodine gel can be applied once or twice daily until the lesions have healed. This medication kills the virus on contact and may help prevent spread of the disease to other areas or to other individuals (see pages 188–90). The drug, acyclovir (Zovirax), available topically and orally, is very useful in suppressing herpes outbreaks. Try to have herpes diagnosed and acyclovir prescribed with the earliest symptoms. Though very expensive, it is the only drug available for herpes sufferers, and has only minimal side effects.

Women who get an initial outbreak of herpes during pregnancy have a higher than average miscarriage rate. There is no good evidence, however, that recurrent herpes during pregnancy increases the risk of spontaneous abortion or premature birth. The concern is that the virus can be passed to the fetus as it passes through an infected birth canal during delivery. Brain damage, blindness, and death occur in the majority of infected babies. Fortunately, herpes infection during birth is rare, occurring in only 1 out of 3,000 live births. If the presence of active internal sores is suspected, a cesarean section may be scheduled. If the sores are present only externally, it may be possible to cover them with a synthetic skin and proceed with a vaginal delivery.

There is increasing evidence that women with herpes sores or genital ulcers are more susceptible to AIDS. Women who have herpes are encouraged to have a Pap smear every six months. This is because researchers suspect a link between herpes and cervical cancer, in which case, routine Pap smears may be very important in the early diagnosis of any abnormal cervical cells.

Atrophic Vaginitis, by definition, is a reaction of the vagina due wholly or in part to a lack of the hormone estrogen. It is not only uncommon but the majority of women who do have an atrophic vagina are completely free of symptoms. The three times in a woman's life when the vagina is atrophic are before the initial onset of menstruation, while breast-feeding, and after menopause.

Typical symptoms include vaginal soreness and occasional spotting. There may be itching and a watery discharge, and intercourse may be painful. As the body's supply of estrogen diminishes, the vaginal walls become thinner and more susceptible to infection. Symptoms are almost exclusively found in women who are well into menopause or who have had their ovaries removed.

Treatment includes using vaginal lubricants during intercourse (sterile lubricants can be bought at drugstores, but you can also try pure vegetable oils or coconut oil from the health food store). Topical estrogen, oral estrogen, or testosterone can also be helpful in alleviating the condition.

Cervicitis is a term used to describe an inflammation or infection of the cervix. It may or may not be anything to worry about, depending on the specific nature of the problem. Varying with the severity and length of infection, there may be a white or cloudy yellow-tan discharge exuding from the endocervical glands. The discharge is not irritating; similarly, there is no soreness, itching, burning, or odor. The cervix may bleed during examination with a speculum or when a Pap smear is performed.

Some forms of cervicitis can cause fertility problems by blocking the route for the sperm to pass and by altering the composition of the cervical fluid so that sperm cannot survive. Other forms may be nothing more than the result of injury of the cervix from childbirth, infection, an IUD, or intercourse; these require no treatment. Some practitioners suggest that women with cervicitis use pads instead of tampons.

Doderlein Cytolysis, an excess of lactobacilli (the good bacteria normally resident in the vagina), is a new culprit in the world of vaginitis and frequently misdiagnosed. Unlike most vaginal problems, doderlein cytolysis is treated by raising the pH of the vagina, often with a sodium bicarbonate solution. Symptoms are discharge and severe itching. The discharge may be either thin and watery or thick and curdlike.

> The physician who relies primarily on the history and gross observation and who tends to ignore the microscopic findings erroneously treats the discharge as recurrent candidiasis. . . . Effective treatment consists of making the vagina more alkaline by douching with distilled water or sodium bicarbonate. Our treatment is one to two tablespoons of bicarbonate in one pint of water as a douche two or three times a week during the symptomatic period.
>
> —Drs. Cibley and Cibley, 1986

Nonspecific Vaginitis is just as its name implies as no causal agent has been identified. It may be due to an outgrowth of normally harmless bacteria in the vagina, unidentified microorganisms, or possibly just to a reaction between the penis and the chemistry of the vagina. It may be the result of intercourse or improper wiping after defecation. Symptoms vary. The discharge is usually odorous and may be gray, white, or yellow, and may possibly be streaked with blood. The vaginal walls can be cloudy, puffy with fluid, and covered by a thick, heavy coat of pus. Itching and burning occur, along with lower back pain, cramps, and swollen groin glands. Treatment for nonspecific vaginitis varies according to specific symptoms. Vinegar douches can be used to maintain the proper acidity of the vagina.

Vaginitis is more common when a woman is sexually active; each new partner increases the odds of developing vaginal symptoms. Sexual activity is only one of the associated factors, for nutrition, stress, age, contraceptive method, and menstrual side effects have also been incriminated. Try and identify the triggers for you.

Guidelines for Avoiding Vaginitis

There are a handful of basic guidelines to follow to reduce your chances of getting vaginitis:

- Women are more likely to have infections when they have a new partner, or when they have more than one partner. Using condoms in the early stages with a new partner, and any time you have more than one partner, is your best bet for protecting yourself. It is also the only available protection against AIDS.
- Don't have intercourse if you have any symptoms of infection. You may be able to avoid transmitting an infection to your partner. If you have itching, redness, pain, or an unusual discharge,

intercourse may be uncomfortable and may make your symptoms worse.

- Not treating the problem or treating the wrong problem will only allow the infection to get worse and possibly increase the risk of having it spread through your reproductive tract. A correct diagnosis is essential.

- Your partner may need to be treated at the same time as you. With many infections, the likelihood of reinfection is great unless all partners are treated simultaneously. Sometimes partners do not have clear symptoms of infections, but should be treated nonetheless. (You cannot assume he or she is infection-free.) Use condoms until you are certain both you and your partner(s) have been cured.

- If you get a prescription from your doctor, use all the medicine. With many drugs, especially antibiotics, you should use the full course even though symptoms may have subsided. If you are using a home treatment, continue the remedy for a few extra days once the symptoms have subsided.

There are some very useful books to have around the house for general gynecological information and care. A list of these can be found in Appendix C. Every home should have at least one of these as a reference guide.

Yeast Infections as Indicators of Other Problems

Because yeast infections tend to be secondary infections, the fact that a stubborn yeast problem exists may be an indicator of some deeper health concerns. Since some weakness in our bodies (the primary health problem) had to be present in order for the yeast overgrowth to have developed, the existence of the infection is a sign that we should examine our overall lifestyle. In that sense, the yeast infection can serve as a diagnostic tool in helping us approach previously unsuspected medical conditions.

But is it possible for the Candida to be more than an indicator of a deeper health issue? Could the Candida population itself be wreaking havoc on the body? One theory popular in the late 1980s was that internal yeast overgrowth and/or yeast hypersensitivity results in a number of maladies not traditionally associated with fungal invasion.

Diaper rash, ringworm, athlete's foot, eczema, yeast vaginitis, oral thrush, and tinea ungium (a common fungal infection of the finger- and toenails) are diseases known to be caused by the yeast organism. Over the last decade, a few researchers and authors proposed a new hypothesis that overgrowth of Candida organisms throughout the body and a hypersensitivity to those organisms was responsible for a host of maladies not traditionally thought to have any connection to yeast whatsoever. The basic theory is that large colonies of yeast release toxins in the body which get absorbed into the bloodstream. The increased number of antigens and toxins in the blood overwhelms the immune system cells, reducing your degree of immunity. This lowered ability to fight diseases leaves you susceptible to a myriad of symptoms and disorders. Various names have been given to this syndrome; one of the more popular is *Polysystemic Chronic Candidiasis* (PSCC).

Some of the maladies attributed to PSCC include: acne, allergies, anxiety, asthma, chemical sensitivity, constipation, depression, diarrhea, earaches, erratic sleep patterns, fatigue, headaches, heartburn, hyperactivity, infertility, irrational irritability, lethargy, loss of sex drive, muscle weakness, poor appetite, poor mem-

There are many versions of a PSCC quiz designed to help identify those people most likely to suffer from yeast-related illness. Questions usually look for affirmative answers on the following types of issues:

- current or past use of antibiotics, birth control pills, and/or cortisone drugs;
- medical conditions that have evaded diagnosis or cure;
- dietary habits high in refined carbohydrates, cravings for sweets, alcohol, or yeast-containing foods (bread, cheese, mushrooms, etc.);
- multiple pregnancies;
- persistent fungal infections (athlete's foot, eczema, vaginitis);
- chemical sensitivity; and
- mood swings or depression (especially on damp days or around moldy places).

ory, persistent coughs, premenstrual syndrome, recurrent vaginitis, spastic colon, and skin irritations.

PSCC has caused a considerable amount of controversy in the medical profession. According to John Bennett of the National Institutes for Health, "Few illnesses have sparked as much hostility between the medical community and a segment of the lay community as the chronic candidiasis syndrome." There is very little data on the incidence of PSCC and none on the percentage of vaginal yeast infection sufferers who also fit the clinical picture of PSCC. Critics say that while the syndrome has appeal (who hasn't suffered from at least a few of the suspected symptoms), and while it is possible that the symptoms are connected in some way, this yeast link is seriously lacking in scientific evidence. They maintain that all aspects of PSCC are speculative and unproven and that the remedies proposed do not withstand scientific scrutiny.

One source of confusion about PSCC stems from the fact that there are no reliable tests to measure it. A study done in 1990 found that a placebo was just as effective as the medication (oral nystatin) in relieving systemic symptoms. Critics argue that desperate people are forced to undergo a rigorous and possibly hazardous treatment regimen in the hopes of curing a disorder that doesn't exist.

PSCC proponents don't deny the lack of quantitative measurements, acknowledging that there are, as yet, no reliable tests to verify the suspected diagnosis of PSCC. "Unlike most infections and infestations, it is not really possible to test for the presence of Candida to prove or disprove such an assumption," explains Leon Chaitow, author of *Candida Albicans*. "The way to prove that a condition (or a cluster of conditions) is the result of Candida is to treat it, and if the symptoms disappear, the proof is irrefutable." Hundreds of practitioners from California to Maine have done just that with reported successes.

The controversy over whether yeast hypersensitivity even exists continues, but the popularity of the theory has waned. There is no question that in women who are suffering from chronic vaginal candidiasis, there is an existing problem with yeast. If you have no other medical concerns besides the vaginal candidiasis, it makes no difference whether PSCC exists or not—you simply treat your condition. If you also suffer from some of the other maladies associated with PSCC, however, you may want to explore the PSCC theory with your physician. The treatments (described below) are more difficult than dangerous. Proponents claim that results should be noticeable within a month, so it doesn't take long to try it.

Treatment consists of a two-faceted approach. The

first is the use of oral antifungals. Nystatin is most commonly used. Caprylic acid is an over-the-counter alternative (see chapter 5 for more information on these). Secondly, some practitioners prescribe a highly restricted diet designed to reduce the intake of foods on which yeast can grow as well as to eliminate any foods which they claim can trigger an allergic reaction or hypersensitivity response. Although there are several variations on the diet, generally the anti-Candida diet requires the elimination of all sugars and highly processed foods as well as any foods containing yeast, including anything with mold or fungus as an ingredient. This encompasses: all bread and breaded foods; beer, wine, and other alcoholic beverages; hard cheeses; mushrooms; dried or smoked meats; and most condiments (mustard, mayonnaise, soy sauce, vinegar, ketchup, pickles, etc.). More information on the diet can be found at the end of chapter 6. However, these diets have not been scrutinized or evaluated for safety and effectiveness. Other common recommendations are to avoid damp, moldy places and to minimize exposure to chemicals.

The best way to fully understand the theories and treatments for this syndrome is to study one or more of the books devoted to the subject listed in Appendix C. If they are not in stock at your local bookstore or health food store, ask the merchant to order a copy for you.

4

❧

WHEN SHOULD YOU GO TO A DOCTOR?
The Physical and Emotional Aspects of Yeast Infections

•

I've had yeast infections every month for so long now, I'd have to be out of my mind to go to a doctor each time. All they ever do is charge a lot of money and give me Monistat. It's just not worth it to bother.

—31-year-old from New York

The last time I thought I had a yeast infection I used some leftover Gyne-Lotrimin, but it didn't work. Finally, I decided to see my doctor. It turned out to be gardnerella (I'd never even heard of that before!). Now I see the doctor anytime anything is wrong. It just seems like the responsible thing to do.

—37-year-old from St. Paul

These women express two different views on the question many women ask: "Should I go to the doctor every time I think I have a yeast infection?" The answer is not a clear yes or no because each woman faces different circumstances and has a different history.

If you do have a yeast infection, but postpone treatment, it may get worse; it will not, however, lead to any permanent damage. Your medical history and your approach to medical care, in general, will largely determine whether you pick up the phone and make an appointment. *But if you are not suffering from a yeast infection, or if you have multiple infections, postponing medical attention and prompt treatment may pose serious risk—to your health and your fertility.* A wise decision requires knowledge about the many vaginal pathogens and their associated risks. (See chapter 3 for a discussion of these.)

The biggest risk in not going to a doctor is that you might have something other than, or in addition to, a yeast infection. A 1984 article helps illustrate this point:

> It was surprising that of two hundred fifty women with alleged chronic recurrent vulvovaginal candidiasis referred to my laboratory over the last year by gynecologists and family practitioners or by self-referral, only one-third were found to have Candida vaginitis. Thus, a patient's failure to respond to treatment may often be the result of the physician's failure to confirm the diagnosis.
>
> —Dr. Jack Sobel, *Annals of Internal Medicine*

Similarly, a British gynecologist explains:

> Not all itchy vaginal discharge is caused by Candida and indeed not all vaginal candidosis is invariably itchy. Without a reasonably accurate diagnosis the treatment is destined to fail in more cases than

necessary thus leading to misunderstanding and patient dissatisfaction.

—Dr. P. J. H. Tooley, *The Practitioner*

The general term for any of many reproductive tract problems involving irritation or inflammation of the vagina is *vaginitis*. Until you know what troubles you, all you know is that you have some form of vaginitis. As we saw in chapter 3, there are no conclusive tests for yeast infections; diagnosis has more to do with the presence of symptoms and the absence of other disease entities. Understandably, it would be useful to have some criteria in deciding when to seek professional help.

Many women who are chronic sufferers of yeast infection find that there is no need to pay a visit to the doctor each time a new infection hits. It only wastes time and money to confirm something they already know.

> When I was in college, I got used to going to the clinic every time I got an infection. They would look at me and give me a sample tube of Monistat to take home. It wasn't until I got out of college and had to start paying for my visits that I realized how expensive it was. After paying for three or four office visits, lab tests, and prescriptions, I gave that up. Every time I'd go, they'd tell me I had a yeast infection. Now I save the money and treat myself with vinegar douches and yogurt; it's as effective as the Monistat ever was.
>
> —29-year-old stockbroker

As reviewed in chapter 3, if vaginitis is present, yet you feel confident that it is a yeast infection just like the ones you've had before and nothing in your life has changed much, and you are not pregnant, there may be no reason to look further than your medicine chest and drug or health food store. But, you must seek medical consultation if:

- you have had only a few yeast infections and are really not sure whether the current infection is the same type as the earlier ones;
- you have a new sexual partner, you have multiple partners, or your sexual partner(s) have new partners;
- you have any symptoms of anything other than those associated with a classic yeast infection (see page 1);
- you feel you have a classic yeast infection, but the treatments which have always worked before aren't working;
- you are confident that you have a yeast infection, but prefer to use prescription treatments and cannot get a prescription without seeing a medical doctor;
- you've recently gone through a physiological change, i.e., puberty, pregnancy, menopause.

What to Expect

When you seek help from a medical professional, what can you expect? First, you'll want to review your present condition and your medical history. Tell him/her what form of birth control you use (if any), when you began your last menstrual cycle, if you are or have recently taken any medication (especially antibiotics or immunosuppressants), if you are sexually active, and review your history of vaginitis (and treatments). You should expect to have a pelvic exam, a Pap smear, and a "wet mount." Request these if the practitioner has not already decided to do them.

If you are going to the doctor and suspect you will be having a pelvic exam, do not douche, medicate, have intercourse, or use any vaginal products for 48 hours preceding the visit. All these things can mask the true clinical picture.

A pelvic exam provides the clinician with a chance to examine your vaginal region visually for any signs of infection. They will be looking at the type and quantity of discharge, swelling, and signs of general irritation. A complete checkup will include an intravaginal examination: The clinician, wearing a plastic glove, inserts one or more fingers into your vagina searching for anything that feels abnormal and trying to locate any area where you may be experiencing pain or tenderness.

The clinician will then generally do a Pap smear, a test that looks for cancerous or abnormal cells on the cervix. The test involves inserting a speculum into the vagina (a speculum is a metal or plastic device, shaped roughly like a hollow squirt gun, that holds the vaginal lips open) then inserting a small (wooden or plastic) spatula, a large Q-tip or small brush to gently scrape a thin layer of cells from the cervix. The cells are then placed on a clean glass slide so they can be microscopically studied at a laboratory.

Cervical cancer is the second most prevalent cancer in women (breast cancer tops the list), and Pap smears are the best screening tests for detecting the cell changes that may precede cancer early enough for appropriate and effective treatment. The incidence of cervical cancer increases with age. If caught early enough, it is fully curable. Studies have shown that women who do not have routine Pap tests develop this disease two to four times more than women who receive regular screening. Two caveats: results may be

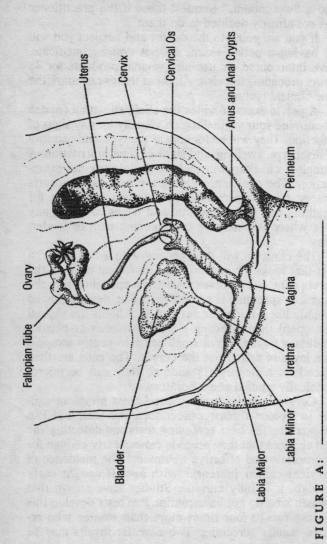

FIGURE A:

Cross-sectional view of female pelvis

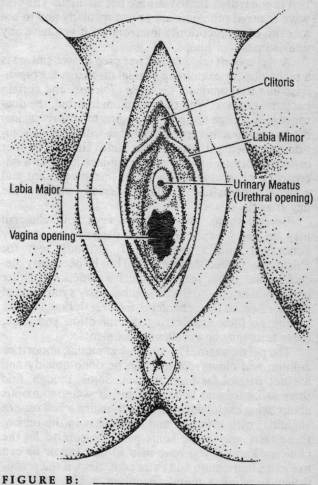

Clitoris

Labia Minor

Labia Major

Urinary Meatus
(Urethral opening)

Vagina opening

FIGURE B:

Diagram of vaginal area

less reliable when there is an infection present. If the results are not clear, have a repeat Pap once the infection is gone; also, these tests are not infallible. The best ways to avoid problems are to test regularly and to see a health care practitioner immediately if you have any unusual pains or lumps.

A wet mount (also called wet prep or wet smear) is a technique for examining vaginal discharge for organisms like trichomonas, *Candida albicans,* and certain bacterial entities. With the speculum inserted, the doctor places a large Q-tip in the vagina to absorb vaginal discharge, then mixes the discharge with a saline solution and smears it onto a glass slide. The practitioner or laboratory technician then examines it under a microscope observing which organisms are present and growing successfully. Results are usually available the day after the test.

Beyond these, two additional tests your clinician may do are a separate culture designed to identify gonorrhea and a monoclonal antibody test for chlamydia (called Microtrak). This is necessary because a wet smear is not conclusive evidence of either gonorrhea or chlamydia. If you have any symptoms of either of these (see chapter 3 for descriptions) or are having no luck eradicating the infection you have, these tests may be excellent investments.

The pelvic exam, Pap smear, wet mount, gonorrhea culture, and chlamydia test can be done quickly and are not painful for most women. Some, though, find them awkward and uncomfortable. If you are anxious about being examined or are experiencing a bad case of vaginitis, with irritation and tenderness in the region, these tests may cause some pain. Be sure to let the clinician know if you have pain so that she or he can use extra lubrication and extra care. Also, if the practitioner is using a metal speculum, make sure it is warmed before insertion.

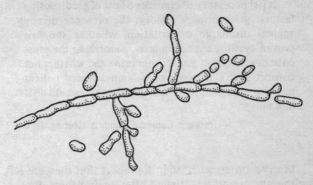

FIGURE C: _____

Under the microscope, candida organisms look like this.

(There are an emerging set of immunological response tests being marketed for use in the diagnosis of Candida. They attempt to measure antibody levels in the body as a way of determining general yeast sensitivity. These tests are quite new, can be costly, and it is unclear whether the information they provide is really useful. At present, there is little indication that they are valuable in diagnosing or treating candidal vaginitis.)

The Traditional Medical Approach

While going to the doctor is often the responsible thing to do, it does not guarantee that you will receive an accurate diagnosis. *A diagnosis for Candida vaginitis is made by reviewing patient history, observing current symptoms, and negative tests for any other disease entity; not by testing positively for yeast.* Accordingly, it takes time and careful analysis to do correctly. Dr. Morton of the Royal Infirmary (Sheffield, England) explains:

It [is] necessary to consider a host of predisposing factors: genitourinary history; the presence of any vaginal discharge or irritation, whether she had proven cystitis, trichomoniasis, gonorrhea; the presence or absence of sugar in her urine and whether her consort had symptoms of balanitis. Every patient must be dealt with individually and no one could do it in a hurry.

—Trends in Candidal Vaginitis Meeting, 1976

Many women with vaginitis report that they are left feeling angry and unsatisfied after seeing their doctor. Their criticisms often include the brief time physicians allocate for each patient, doctors' unwillingness to discuss the diagnosis, an inability to provide anything other than short-term relief, and a condescending attitude toward vaginitis. Dr. Sobel, Chief of Infectious Diseases at Wayne State University, believes:

There is no doubt that when it comes to the diagnosis and treatment of chronic candidiasis, women have been terribly abused. The medical profession, especially gynecologists and family practitioners, have almost no clinical acumen for diagnosing yeast infections. Their whole approach is unacceptably poor and the only reason they get away with it is that nobody dies of chronic candidiasis.

From the lazy physician's point of view, there is almost no harm in diagnosing a patient positive for *Candida albicans*. After all, there is often yeast in the vagina, so it is not necessarily incorrect. Besides, the unnecessary use of the common prescription antifungals aren't likely to cause any harm to anyone.

I remember going to this one doctor for my annual Pap smear. Every time I went he told me I had a yeast infection. I would take his prescription home and put it in my desk drawer figuring if I ever felt like I had an infection, I'd have one filled. My mother always taught me, "if it ain't broke, don't fix it." I never did fill any of them.

—34-year-old lawyer

I went to the doctor last year because I was afraid I had herpes. It turned out to be just a clogged hair follicle. But the doctor told me I had a yeast infection and wrote me out a prescription for Monistat. I knew I didn't have a yeast infection. I think he was just afraid to send me home empty-handed. I was relieved that I didn't have herpes, but was really angry that he told me I had an infection that didn't exist. In retrospect, that whole visit was a waste of time.

—25-year-old in Washington, D.C.

If you have had bad experiences with physicians, it is most likely not because the doctor is stupid, lazy, or malicious. It is, most likely, simply that the doctor does not know enough about Candida vaginitis. This is so for several reasons.

First, Western medicine tends to fit disease entities into a cause and effect scenario (viruses cause colds, bacteria cause bladder infections, vitamin C deficiencies cause scurvy). Yeast vaginitis is viewed similarly. A woman complains of a yeast infection, the doctor cultures yeast from the vaginal fluids, a diagnosis is made: The yeast caused the vaginitis. Because the patient has a vaginal infection, the obvious treatment approach is a vaginal preparation that will eradicate the yeast. Of course, the missing piece of the equation is that the positive culture for yeast does not necessarily tell us anything of significance since yeast can live inside the vagina quite harmlessly.

The Western medical focus, then, revolves around treatment of the vagina and only the vagina (killing the yeast where they have been identified). When treatments fail (which they often do), the medical response is to treat the vagina even more vigorously. The common result is that a patient will be told to use intravaginal antifungals almost continuously or to use antifungals as a prophylactic for the week just before menses every month. In either case, the treatment is inadequate for two reasons: it limits treatment to the vagina, and its success is judged by the momentary elimination of symptoms, even though recurrence is common.

Second, doctors absorb most of their knowledge about any illness in medical school. This training may have been decades ago for your physician(s). Men run the medical schools and, until recently, almost all the students were men. Women's issues (as they were labeled) did not receive the greatest amount of interest or attention. In fact, several studies have discovered widespread medical bias against female patients. In one study, women and men sought medical care with an identical array of symptoms. Doctors showed less concern and ordered fewer follow-up tests for women than they had for men. The high number of unnecessary hysterectomies, mastectomies, and cesareans, as well as the significantly disproportionate share of tranquilizers prescribed to women, have all been attributed to this medical gender bias.

Third, with the huge body of knowledge the students need to digest, some topics receive less emphasis than others. Yeast infections are hardly a source of extended stimulating lectures in medical school. Indeed, they are considered rather mundane, local events that can be easily eradicated by any of a number of safe antifungals. Since nobody dies of vaginal yeast infections, there is very little status or glamour in studying the disease.

Fourth, the incidence and severity of the disease have been dramatically increasing, due largely, as we have seen, to long-term use of antibiotics, immunosuppressants, and oral contraceptives. It takes time for the medical community to recognize, review, revise, and distribute updated information.

Finally, some blame must be shouldered by the pharmaceutical companies. Full-page and multi-page advertisements for anticandida formulations litter the medical journals, and sales reps distribute product samples to physicians to distribute to patients—with a prescription for additional quantities. The ads tout the convenience and efficiency of the formulations in clearing vaginitis, and they proclaim in large letters that studies show their drugs to have low recurrence rates. The small print, however, reveals that they only looked for recurrence two or three weeks after treatment; the interval for recurrence for these products in the manufacturers' studies rarely exceeds four weeks. For the woman who gets six, perhaps eight, yeast infections a year, low recurrence after a few weeks is hardly significant.

With a disease such as yeast vaginitis, the pharmaceutical companies can only profit when their drugs are assumed to be the answer and any resulting recurrence translates into significant additional sales. Conversely, the companies want you and your doctor to believe that since the drugs are proven effective, recurrence could only mean you used an inadequate amount or that the treatment time wasn't long enough. The "cure" these companies want you to have is dependence on their drugs.

Of course, not all doctors are bad and not all drug companies are evil, but the modern medical model has been negligent in addressing the very real problems women are facing with recurrent vulvovaginal candidosis. It would be wonderful if there were a panacea drug that would eradicate once and for all any yeast infection that reared its nasty head; unfortunately, effective treatment is a bit more complex. You, as the patient, need to educate yourself about the illness and be willing to search for a medical practitioner who will work with you to resolve the condition.

Some women who have trouble finding a doctor they feel comfortable with have chosen to go it alone, with self-help books and home remedies. Still others have sought out nontraditional medical care. Midwives, nurse practitioners, nutritionists, and chiropractors can all be effective health care providers for medical doctors are not the only people who can establish a diagnosis and treatment regimen. And, while there is no guarantee that you will find a superb nontraditional health professional, many women do report a high rate of satisfaction with this approach due to these practitioners' higher degree of concern and the significant amount of time and attention they give.

> After about a half-dozen yeast infections, I decided to drop my male general practitioner and find a female gynecologist. She was not only unsympathetic, but didn't appear to know much about yeast infections at all. I was really disappointed. I guess I had just assumed that a woman doctor would be superior. Eventually I heard about a midwife that also provided well-woman care. I've been seeing her for years now; she's just wonderful.
>
> —39-year-old teacher in Virginia

If you chose to see a health practitioner who cannot do pelvic exams and order laboratory tests, remember that regular gynecological care is also an important part of general health care. Make sure you have a medical checkup at least once a year. Exclusively lesbian women may be spared many of the gynecological problems that plague heterosexual and bisexual women, and as such, have fewer gynecological exams. They, for example, average twenty-one months between Pap smears while heterosexual women average one every eight months. All women should have regular gynecological exams that include a Pap smear. The American Cancer Society recommends a Pap at least every three years after two normal annual screenings until the age of sixty-five. However, the American College of Obstetricians and Gynecologists recommends annual Paps, especially for sexually active women. Women with herpes may want to have one done every six months.

The Emotional Chaos

All the chaos surrounding your chronic yeast infections—searching for a good doctor, repeated pelvic exams, messy prescriptions, painful intercourse, and then another infection—exacts more of a toll on you than may be obvious. While there is no question that chronic vaginitis can be physically painful and financially troubling, the emotional cost can equal and even outweigh this. One isolated infection may be nothing more than a nuisance, two in a year inconvenient. But three infections in three months can create tension in your personal relationships, reduce your efficiency at work, and lower your self-esteem. As the itching and burning increases, as the regularity sets in, the psychological toll from repeated infections grows steadily greater.

There is little written about the emotional stress experienced by women suffering from chronic yeast infections in either the medical journals or the women's self-help books. Feelings of frustration and vulnerability are common. You may go from doctor to doctor, from prescription to prescription, without lasting relief. Your partner might accuse you of deliberately getting infections to avoid intimacy while your friends might feel you exaggerate your problems just to draw attention to yourself. Your boss might conclude that you make up medical excuses just to get time off work. The effects of the infections reach far beyond your vagina.

When we were young, we learned that if we got sick, the doctor would make us better. Now that we are adults, we still want the doctor to tell us exactly what is wrong and to provide us a quick fix. Often, this is exactly what happens. But when presented with chronic yeast infections, most traditional medical professionals simply do not have the tools to provide that fix, giving us instead what amounts to a bandage. All the conventional wisdom (medical texts, pharmaceutical advertisements, etc.) suggests that the drugs work and work well. When reinfection occurs, the doctors generally conclude that your case is particularly stubborn and usually prescribe multiple doses of the same medicines. When this, too, proves ineffective, the doctor, out of frustration, might label you psychosomatic, and you, similarly, might label the doctor incompetent. In truth, the fault lies with the medical system's basic lack of understanding about this problem.

> You know what really kills me. There you are, half naked, lying on your back, your legs spread, feet in those cold metal stirrups—the doctor has just spent ten minutes poking around inside you. He takes off his glove, washes his hands, and tells you it's just a

minor irritation. He says, "Women get them all the time, nothing to worry about." He doesn't care. Does he honestly think I would have ended up practically naked in his office if I felt it were a minor infection. He could have at least pretended to care.

—34-year-old woman from Boston

Trying to tell a doctor that the intravaginal creams don't work can be an exercise in frustration. If you complain of recurring infections, the standard medical advice is to use a tube of cream each time you feel an infection coming on, or maybe use two, or maybe use it through your menstrual cycle, or use it for the next couple of weeks. And, if the infection comes back, just get more—there's plenty of refills on the prescription.

After a while, I figured either the doctor owned stock in the company that makes Monistat, or he just didn't know what he was doing. And he wouldn't listen to me. It was obvious the stuff wasn't keeping the infections from coming back. He wanted me to use the cream four weeks out of every month, a proposition I could neither afford or put up with.

—College student in Texas

Everybody always assumed the doctors were right and I was somehow wrong. Like I wasn't using the prescription right or something. It really bugged me that no one believed the medication didn't work, they just assumed that I had screwed up.

—32-year-old school bus driver

Many women have described their friends' reactions to their maladies as being tantamount to "blaming the victim." As if it's not enough to suffer from the physical illness, you also suffer from the insensitive remarks of others. The message behind a statement like, "She must not take very good care of herself if she keeps getting those infections," is that you are responsible for some underlying deficiency in your body. Pretty soon you figure out that it's easier not to discuss the problem with most people. It doesn't take long, under these circumstances, to start to become isolated and withdrawn from those with whom you were once close.

Making matters even worse is the fear and guilt our society associates with illnesses "down there"—on our sex organs. Syphilis and gonorrhea, routine diseases that can be accurately diagnosed and completely cured, are unmentionable words. The subject of herpes can kill any conversation. With the recent concerns over AIDS, this fear has become more extreme. All this leaves the individual feeling it's better to be miserable alone than to risk the embarrassment of telling anyone.

> I used to get yeast infections fairly regularly, two or three times a semester. My boyfriend at the time used to freak out. He would make me feel dirty, like if he got near me, he would "catch" it and his wick would shrivel. Each time I could feel the itching start, I knew that I'd not only have to deal with the infection, but I'd also have to deal with all his carryings-on. I guess it's not surprising that the infections lasted longer than the boyfriend.
>
> —26-year-old in Oregon

The cycle of misunderstanding and lack of compassion often starts in the doctor's office, extends to the partner, and continues from there. People who can usually be counted on to be supportive may be quite critical—perhaps because of the embarrassment they feel talking about sex, perhaps because they feel helpless to do anything about it.

> I think one of the hardest parts for me had to be the hidden messages. My mother and my girlfriends were supportive at first, but after a while, they made me feel like the infections were somehow my fault. They never said anything directly, but it was there. They'd pick easy targets, like implying that if I didn't go out so much, if I wasn't always so busy, if I didn't shower at the gym, I wouldn't get them as often. One friend even stated flatly that my body was telling me to start eating red meat again.
>
> —31-year-old in California

Another issue that may work against you is the belief that you can control everything that happens in your life. For some women, there is a conviction that everything that happens does so because (on some level, unconscious or subconscious) you want or need it to happen.

> After a while, I really began to lose a lot of self-confidence. I had always believed in the power of the mind. That's probably why I got so depressed when my vaginitis didn't go away. I really believed that if I just could get the image of a healthy vagina ingrained in my mind, I would get better. I spent hours meditating on the image of an infection-free body. Instead I just kept getting worse. I couldn't figure out what I had done to deserve this.
>
> —28-year-old Canadian woman

Some women have surprised themselves by discovering feelings of resentment toward other women who don't suffer from yeast infections.

> I hadn't told many people about my infections, but I finally decided to tell one of my friends. I figured it would help me if I started talking about it. She replied almost instantly that she'd never had one and couldn't even imagine what it must be like. I felt this rage start to grow from inside me. It was horrible. All I could think about was that life was unfair and about how much I envied her.
>
> —42-year-old in Cleveland

After a while, it seems like everything is working against you. If specialists treat your vaginitis as trivial, if "proven" pharmaceuticals provide nothing more than temporary relief, if those around you blame you for your illness, if you are made to feel unclean, if you feel distant from your friends—it would almost require superhuman resolve not to feel alone and isolated. Intimate relationships start to erode under the strain.

The lack of an adequate medical solution indicates that a different approach to treatment is needed—as much as it indicates that unresolved feelings need to be resolved. The fact is that many people are able to benefit from counseling. Resolving painful emotional issues may help to improve your general health and may certainly help in dealing with the turmoil the vaginitis has caused. But any work on the emotional issues must be together with work on the physical condition. Since the emotions are not the cause of your problem, they alone cannot be the cure.

Dr. Rosalinde Hurley describes in the British medical journal, *The Practitioner,* what she has observed in her work with women suffering from chronic yeast vaginitis:

> Frequent complaint is made of tearfulness, irritability, marital discord, and foreboding of suicide. Sexual relationships are severely strained; some patients are already divorced or separated, whilst the unmarried attribute their single state, in no small measure, to the persistent vulvovaginitis. . . .
>
> . . . Patients are able to describe not only the symptoms but the signs, since they are habituated to examining themselves with mirrors . . . the pruritus is intense and more or less constant. Patients scratch in an endeavour to obtain relief and the vulva bleeds, becoming excoriated and ulcerated . . . Because of the long history, and the many practitioners consulted, it is often difficult to date the onset of symptoms accurately.
>
> . . . Above all, the patients must be dissuaded from the notion that they represent a class of medical freaks.

Fortunately, there can be an end to this private cycle of pain. It won't be handed to you on a silver platter, nor will it produce instantaneous results. But it can help you regain and retain a vital, healthy life—free from infection and all its associated worries.

The first step in getting well is understanding both the problem and the approach to treatment. And remember, you are not alone. Yeast infections afflict millions of women. The more you share with and learn from others, the better. Reading and talking to other people is important. You will be amazed at how many women you already know have been going through the same thing as you. There is almost nothing better for the soul than talking with people who have suffered through the same problems.

> At first I was just depressed. All I could think of was how long it would be until the next infection. Once I started learning about yeast and practicing prevention, everything changed. I haven't had a yeast infection in over a year now and the difference in me is like night and day. I no longer expect to be sick, I've stopped feeling like I had no control over my life. I still don't like to remember what it was like, I'm just so grateful to be rid of those awful infections.
>
> —28-year-old swimming coach

With an understanding of the yeast organism, appropriate treatment, and a healthy lifestyle, you will soon reach the moment when chronic, painful, vaginal yeast infections are nothing more than a bad chapter from your past.

※

•

PART TWO

•

TREATING YEAST

•

※

To thee only I appeal, Not to thy noble son,
whose yeasty youth Will clear itself, and crystal turn again.

—Keats

5

❧

GETTING FREE

•

> Treatment of the yeast problem seeks not the eradication of yeast from the diet or the person, but rather a new relationship between the person and the yeast.
>
> —Dr. Sidney Baker, Notes on the Yeast Problem

*T*his chapter is about achieving goals. The short-term goal is eradication of discharge, itching, and irritation, that is, clearing up the yeast infection. This is not a terribly difficult problem because any number of widely available formulations can successfully ease your symptoms and eliminate the discomfort. The long-term goal is solving the problem of recurrence, clearing up the infection and its symptoms once and for all.

The difference between stopping one infection and getting rid of the problem altogether is the difference between treatment and cure, between resolving the short-term problem and removing the long-term problem altogether. This chapter presents a four-point program designed to achieve both treatment and cure. Through this four-point strategy, you will learn both general health measures and specific therapies to accomplish a lasting cure.

Four-Point Yeast Eradication Program:

1. Strengthen your overall health
2. Build up yeast-controlling bacteria
3. Reduce the yeast population in the vagina
4. Reduce the yeast population of the gastrointestinal tract

As you begin working the program, think of yourself as a scientist trying to track down the missing pieces of a mystery. You are your own research specimen. Buy a little notebook and use it to jot down thoughts and observations. Start by recording your level (and sources) of stress, your standard meals and snacks, your sexual activity (and type of birth control), any medications taken (especially antibiotics), as well as whether any discharge or itching is present. Do this once a week and be sure to date each entry. Each body is unique and this will give you some indications of what it is that affects your body. Any time you have an increase in itching or discharge, make an entry in your notebook. Did you eat differently, enjoy a new lover, have a sleepless night, or fight with your boss? Only by careful observations of yourself will the missing pieces be solved. You are with yourself 24 hours a day, no one is better equipped to piece together what triggers infections in you. Keep track of what you consume, who you are with, your moods, your level of stress/relaxation, your menstrual cycles, anything that will make it easier to evaluate changes in your vaginal health and to determine what factors are triggering problems for you. It is also a good morale booster to look back as you progress and see how well you're doing.

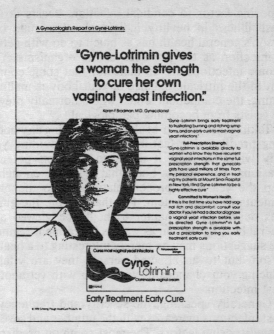

FIGURE D: _____

This ad represents one of the many non-prescription products available that are useful in alleviating immediate vaginal discomfort.

Point One: Strengthen Your Overall Health

Yeast organisms are normally present in the healthy body. While they sometimes cause disease, the factors that transform them from harmless residents to disease entities appear to have more to do with the individual than with the yeast organism itself. From the earliest observations, it has been clear that ill health or physiological change in the patient is the primary predisposing factor to candidal infection. Yeasts do not cause illness in healthy individuals. The state of a person's general health has as much to do with getting an infection as the presence of the organisms. Your chronic infections are an indicator that some component in the intricate balance of your body is malfunctioning, the component which would normally prevent the yeasts from becoming pathological.

Taking care of your health and removing any underlying predisposing factors is key to providing your body with the tools it needs to ward off potential invasions. You want a body that is strong enough to keep the yeasts in proper relationship to the other elements in your system. For that reason, the guidelines described in chapter 6 should be viewed as a general health program as well as a treatment regimen. The suggestions may be merely interesting to a healthy person, but to an affected person, they are vital to reducing your chances of waking up with yet another yeast infection.

Generally speaking, the severity and frequency of yeast infections increases with the number and severity of predisposing factors. The most common predisposing factors are:

- Pregnancy
- Antibiotics
- Birth control pills
- Menstruation
- Cortisone and cortisonelike medications
- Stresses and weaknesses in the immune system
- Nutritional imbalances
- Transmission to/from a sexual partner
- Irritations and abrasions in the vaginal region

The discussion of these in chapter 2 can help you better understand and manage factors that may be contributing to your recurrent yeast infections. If eliminating triggers clears up your infection for the long term, consider yourself lucky. If, however, you are one of the numerous women who finds that infections are repeat visitors, it will just be the first step in your total yeast program.

Point Two: Build Up Your Yeast-Controlling Bacteria

Throughout your intestines and vagina, yeasts and bacteria live together harmoniously. They not only live side-by-side peacefully, but actually work together in an intricate effort to maintain proper functioning of the digestive and vaginal tracts. Normally, this checks-and-balances mechanism occurs without any intervention. However, if the yeast/bacteria ratio is disturbed, the yeast population can grow unchecked. When this occurs, a little intervention can go a long way.

There are several ways to upset the yeast/bacteria balance. Antibiotics, for example, in their zeal to kill illness-causing bacteria, wipe out the helpful intestinal bacteria, too. All antibiotics (the broad-spectrum ones and the tetracyclines especially) dramatically reduce the resident lactobacilli bacterial population of the intestine. The eradication of these yeast-controlling bacteria allows the yeasts to grow unchecked, and they multiply wildly in an all-out effort to cover the membrane surfaces of the intestinal and vaginal tracts.

One clear sign that the intestinal balance has been disturbed is digestive disruption, a common side effect of taking antibiotics. While taking antibiotics is the easiest way to throw off the intestinal mechanisms, it is not the only way. If you have regular gas, bloating, or constipation, it may be an indication that your bacterial population is struggling. Many women who complain of frequent yeast infections also complain of digestive disturbances, not realizing that they may be related.

The normal lactobacilli bacteria that populate the body constitute your single most important natural defense against Candida infections. With a strong lactobacilli population, your body's normal flora defends you against infection by microorganisms. Not surprisingly, patients with vaginal yeast infections have been found to host decreased lactobacilli populations.

The lactobacilli maintain a complex interaction that, in a healthy woman, routinely inhibits pathogenic organisms. They not only actively inhibit fungal growth, but are key to influencing both the quantity and quality of organisms present in the vagina. The bacteria actually compete against the yeasts in your body for glucose. Healthy bacteria will win out over the yeasts for these sugars; hence the yeast is kept in check by the limited growth-promoting nourishment.

As part of their normal course of events, the lactobacilli produce lactic acid and hydrogen peroxide. It is the lactic acid component that is responsible for the normally low vaginal pH. The low pH, in turn, encourages the growth of more lactobacilli organisms, while discouraging the growth of other microorganisms. The hydrogen peroxide also helps inhibit the growth of microorganisms. Finally, it appears that the bacteria themselves have qualities which specifically inhibit fungal growth. Studies have shown that, when cells were precoated with lactobacilli, yeast could not attach themselves to the cell surfaces. Actively promoting lactobacilli growth in your body is probably the easiest and best natural defense against yeast.

One way to promote bacterial growth is to help repopulate the intestines and vagina with "good" bacterial organisms through the consumption of active acidophilus cultures. Acidophilus is a type of "good" bacterium that can be purchased in health food stores.

Promoting good bacteria can be just as important in restoring and maintaining health as eliminating disease-causing microorganisms. Placing acidophilus in the vagina (intravaginal use) will help repopulate the vaginal bacterial population, inhibiting the yeast where they are causing you the most trouble. Adding lactobacilli to your diet may not only reduce your yeast population, but may also reduce the chances of vaginal contamination of yeasts from the rectum.

Acidophilus organisms are actually alive. Commercially, acidophilus are the bacterial organisms that companies use to turn milk into yogurt. Food sources of lactobacilli include yogurt and miso (an oriental soy bean paste). For you, they can supplement and nourish your body's own lactobacilli population. Acidophilus preparations are available in a variety of forms (liquids and tablets are most common), are entirely safe to take, and can be purchased at any health food store. The pills are tasteless, the liquids taste a bit like yogurt. Unless the label specifies that room temperature is acceptable, keep all acidophilus preparations refrigerated.

Acidophilus can be taken by mouth, where the goal is to get it into the intestines, as well as placed directly in the vagina to promote the bacterial population of the vagina. In the beginning of any yeast treatment program, it should be taken orally and used intravaginally. Oral use should continue for two-to-three months in order to ensure that the body's bacteria are increased for a long enough time to maintain a healthy population. Once a healthy environment is stabilized, occasional use may be all that you need for maintenance.

The potency of acidophilus products varies dramatically. Ratings are generally provided on each product by the number of live organisms, for instance, 2.8 billion live organisms per capsule. Generally, the higher the potency, the more you are helping your body. Since acidophilus is most useful where the most yeasts reside—the large and small intestines—and because digestive juices in the stomach can render ineffective some of the acidophilus you swallow, the best way to spend your acidophilus dollars is to buy it in a form which is "enterically coated," that is, prepared in such a way that active cultures pass through the stomach intact.

Acidophilus tablets should be taken on an empty stomach. Powders can be mixed in juice or just added on top of your food. (Do not mix it with seltzer water—it causes a slightly explosive reaction.) Liquid preparations can be taken as is or mixed in milk or juice. Follow the recommended dosage guidelines on the package to determine the amount to take each time. For the first four-to-six weeks, take acidophilus twice a day; for the second two-to-four weeks, once a day should suffice.

Acidophilus organisms are living and keep best under refrigeration (Kyo-Dophilus uses a heat-stable strain that does fine at room temperature, making it a good choice for travelers). Acidophilus should never be frozen. The bacteria are typically grown on a dairy base so people with dairy sensitivities should ask for a brand grown on a vegetable base.

These bacteria are dependent on vitamin B for their growth and cannot survive in an environment without it. A vitamin B-rich diet (e.g., liver, seafood, chicken, eggs, brewer's yeast) will ensure that you have the nutrients you need. An additional vitamin B supplement should also be taken to help promote the growth of lactobacilli. Take one tablet of a balanced vitamin B complex supplement every day with a meal when you are taking acidophilus.

Intravaginal use of acidophilus can be an effective tool in promoting vaginal health and can be a potent weapon in your arsenal of anti-yeast treatments. In one study, reported in 1986, women with vaginitis (yeast as well as other types) were treated by douching twice daily with an acidophilus solution and taking a vitamin B complex supplement. Using this simple treatment regime, 82 percent of the women overcame their infections during the 14-day treatment period. Douches can be helpful in treating vaginitis, including Candida; however, in cases of severe infection an initial stronger medication may be required. In the study cited above, some of the Candida patients with severe infection found the treatment was only effective when supplemented initially with an antifungal.

When there is itching and discharge due to vaginal yeasts, local acidophilus can serve as a very effective remedy. One way to apply acidophilus intravaginally is to pierce one or two capsules (either purchased or homemade using acidophilus powder with empty gelatin capsules) with a pin to create multiple punctures and insert the perforated capsules deeply into the vagina at bedtime. Depending on the specific capsules you use, they will either dissolve or break open allowing the acidophilus to coat the mucous membranes (undissolved empty capsules will simply be expelled with the morning urine). Alternatively, you can also prepare a douche by mixing the contents of two capsules, a half teaspoon of acidophilus powder, or two tablespoons of acidophilus liquid into a pint of warm water. Start treating yourself with acidophilus as soon as vaginal symptoms begin and for two days after they cease. As with all intravaginal treatments, intravaginal acidophilus should only be used for symptomatic relief, not as a routine practice. Do not use any intravaginal treatment for more than fourteen days.

An alternative to intravaginal acidophilus capsules is to insert plain yogurt in the vagina at night. This messy, but less expensive substitute, can be done in many ways. Some women dip a small tampon (O.B.

brand is often used for this) in yogurt, then insert it. Because you may forget to take the tampon out after a few hours, a preferable technique is to use a spermicide-refill or Monistat applicator filled with diluted yogurt. Dilute the yogurt with warm water or a water/vinegar mix (just enough so you can pour it into the applicator or suction it up), and apply the mixture at bedtime. Wear a sanitary pad. Another technique is to use diluted yogurt as a douche mixture.

Antibiotics are designed to kill bacteria, so anytime you plan to take a course of antibiotics, while you are taking them, and for a few days after, it is a good idea to supplement the restoration of "good" bacteria in your intestinal tract (and in your vagina if you are especially prone to yeast infections) with acidophilus. This safe, tasty, and easy-to-use dietary supplement can go a long way toward warding off yeast infections and promoting a healthy vagina.

Acidophilus Resource List

Enterically coated capsules:
   Primadophilus by Nature's Way, 100 capsules for $14.95

Powders:
   Megadophilus by Natren, 2.5 ounces for $17.90
   Primadophilus by Klaire Labs, 2 ounces for $19.95

Liquids:
   Theradophilus, strawberry formula, 8 ounces for $5.49

Nondairy Acidophilus:
   Natren Milk-Free Powder, 2.5 ounces for $17.99
   Kyo-Dophilus, 90 capsules for $16.99

Vitamin B Complex Supplements:
   Solgar, 50 capsules for $3.50
   Twinlab, 100 capsules for $9.95

For more information, see:

Chapter 2, Yeast Triggers (Predisposing Factors)
Chapter 5, Getting Free (Douching)
Chapter 6, Staying Free (Guide to Taking Antibiotics)

Point Three: Reduce the Yeast Population in the Vagina

While the ultimate goal is not to destroy all the yeast organisms in your vagina, the treatment program aims to reduce that population, moving you along the road to recovery. The standard medical method aims to eradicate the yeasts from the vagina using medications that destroy the yeast organisms on contact. For the woman who finds herself with only an occasional, mild infection, this alone may be sufficient. If you have frequent and severe infections, however, this will be just one step in the four-step yeast management program.

There are a plethora of suggested methods to reduce your vaginal yeast and rid yourself of the infection. The home remedies section (later in this chapter) covers over a half dozen inexpensive techniques for arresting yeast infections. The antifungal agents section (still later) lists a variety of prescription and nonprescription methods that also effectively accomplish this goal. While all these are safe and reported to be effective, generally speaking, the antifungal agents appear to work faster, but cost significantly more, than the home remedies. The main criterion in choosing how you approach the problem is simply personal preference.

Point Four: Reduce the Yeast Population of the Gastrointestinal Tract

> . . . that the presence of yeasts in the genital tract is often associated with their presence in the digestive tract . . . lends support to those who advocate treatment of the intestinal tract in patients with chronic symptomatic vulvovaginitis.
>
> —Drs. Hilton and Warnock,
> *British Journal of Obstetrics and Gynecology*

The common view is that candida vaginitis is a simple infection caused by an overgrowth of a single pathogen at a superficial site and that an abundance of very convenient, very effective courses of antifungal therapy exist. Advertisements in medical journals touting the effectiveness of anticandidal drugs lead you to believe that you could be simply and completely cured within a matter of days. However, studies have shown over and over again that none of the standard vaginal treatments have more than a 90 percent primary cure rate and that relapse rates as high as 50 percent are common.

What the pharmaceutical companies promise—and deliver—is relief of acute symptoms. However, long-term relief requires a more extensive yeast management program, one in which treatment is not considered successful until symptoms do not return months after it has ceased.

Women and health practitioners who have learned the hard way the difference between the relief of symptoms and the long-term eradication of the illness have looked more deeply into other forms of treatment. Since the main reservoir of yeast organisms in the body is the lower intestine, recent thought has focused on that area as a possible source for reinfection of the vagina.

The prevalence of Candida organisms is greater in the intestines than it is in either the vagina or the mouth. As the gut harbors the largest concentration of fungi, a number of researchers have determined that, indeed, women with candida vulvovaginitis have greater populations of yeasts in the gastrointestinal tract than women without yeast infections. They have also found that the strain of yeast found in the vagina is the same as that in the individual's gastrointestinal tract.

A comprehensive treatment program seeks to minimize the influence of yeasts in the body as well as minimize the likelihood of yeasts colonizing the vagina. Paying attention to the gastrointestinal tract can help us do both. Applying an antifungal cream around the anus may help reduce the spread of yeasts from the rectum to the vulva and vagina. A study by Forssman and Lars found that such prophylactic treatment reduced significantly recolonization of the vagina. Any prescription antifungal cream or a boric acid ointment can be used for this.

In stubborn cases, taking oral antifungal medication can also be beneficial. There is some controversy over whether one should take these drugs, and for how long, to treat candida vulvovaginitis, but oral nystatin and oral caprylic acid have been shown to be effective at removing yeasts from the gut. Studies have demonstrated that use of oral antifungals reduces the yeast population in the gastrointestinal tract and can be a useful tool in the effort to end recurrent infection. (Nystatin, a prescription antifungal, and caprylic acid, an over-the-counter antifungal, are discussed in detail further in this chapter in the antifungal agents section.)

Researchers have performed a number of studies using simultaneous treatment with oral and topical antifungals. In one study performed by the Nystatin Multicenter Study Group (involving gynecologists in six different countries), it was found that the response rate of the patient population who received combined local-oral therapy was consistently superior to those receiving only local therapy. A 1982 study comparing the effectiveness of six treatment regimens for vulvovaginal candidiasis with six months' follow-up found that the most successful treatment was miconazole vaginal cream with oral nystatin.

There have been studies of oral treatment with less positive results. However, it is unclear whether the mixed results indicate the inaccuracy of the theory or the inadequacy of the oral treatment regime. Some studies used small amounts of nystatin, in others oral nystatin was prescribed for only one week. Longer periods of sustained use seem to be necessary for the highest efficacy.

Nystatin can be taken orally in either tablet or liquid form. You can take ready-made prescription tablets (Nystex or Nilstat) or can make your own capsules using pure prescription nystatin powder. Similarly, ready-made prescription liquids are available or you can mix pure nystatin prescription powder in water or juice. Aside from being easier to take, an additional benefit of tablets is that, if enterically coated, they will have a maximum response in the intestine.

If you want to use the powder, be sure to get pure nystatin powder—not topical powder which consists mostly of talc. If it is not available in a local pharmacy, one source is Freeda Pharmacy, 36 East 41st Street, NY, NY 10017, 800-777-3737. You must have a prescription to get it. Either have your physician call it in on their toll-free number or mail or fax the prescription to them. They will mail the nystatin to you.

Some tips on the powder: usual adult dosage is ¼ to ½ teaspoon (⅛ teaspoon is 500,000 IUs) taken with the same frequency as the tablets (see page 147). It has a distinctly foul taste and is most palatable when mixed with either grapefruit or grape juice. Nystatin should be taken with meals. Prices for nystatin are listed on page 176.

While it is widely agreed that both nystatin and caprylic acid have no side effects, you may experience nausea, especially in the first two weeks. This reaction is called a Herxheimer reaction, which some physicians feel is caused by yeast "die-off"—dead yeast toxins suddenly being released into the body. It is seen not as a side effect (something that happens in addition to the action of the drug), but as proof that the drug is working. If you feel nauseous, cut your intake by half for a few days, then gradually work back up to full dosage.

Caprylic Acid tablets are available in health food stores. There are many brands available, some with just caprylic acid, others combined with vitamins and/or other antifungal agents. Check with your health food store for a caprylic acid formulation. They typically contain 100 mg of caprylic acid per tablet.

Recommended Oral Treatment:

Nystatin (500,000 IU tablets) or Caprylic Acid (100 mg tablets)

2 tablets, 2 times daily (with meals) for 1 month, followed by 1 tablet, 2 times daily (with meals) for 2 months.

Caprylic Acid Resource List:

- Caprystatin, Ecological Formulas, 90 tablets, $18.95
- Mycostat, P & D Nutrition, 90 capsules, $18.10
- Caprinex, Nature's Way, 100 capsules, $11.95
- Capricin, Professional Specialties, 100 capsules, $16.95

SUBSTANCES USED FOR TREATING
YEAST INFECTIONS
(Those with an * are discussed in this book.)

Acidophilus*
Aloe Vera*
Arginine
Barley
Beeswax
Bentonite
Bifidobacteria
Boric Acid*
Burows Solution*
Calendula
  Cream*
Calcium
Caprylic Acid*
Chlorophyll
Cloves
Coenzyme Q10
Egg White
Eucalyptus Oil
Evening Primrose
  Oil
Folic Acid
Garlic*
Gentian Violet*
Ginger Root
Horseradish
Hydrochloric
  Acid
Iron
Lemon*
Linseed Oil
Magnesium
Menthol
Nat. Phos 6X
  (a tissue salt)
Oat Bran
Olive Oil
Onion

Pancreati
Peppermint Oil
Potassium
  Sorbate*
Povidone-Iodine*
Primrose Oil
Propolis
Red Clover
Safflower Oil
Salt*
Selenium
Sodium
  Bicarbonate
Sorbic Acid*
Taheebo (also
  called La
  Pacho or Pau
  D'Arco)
Vinegar*
Vitamin A
Vitamin B
  Formulations*
Vitamin C
Vitamin D
Vitamin E
Wheat Bran
Wheat Germ
Wheat Grass
  Juice
Yeast
  Vaccinations
Yogurt*
Zinc
Zymex Wafers

Herbs:
Agrimony

Barberry Root
Bark
Bladderwrack
Borage
Buckthorn Bark
Capsicum Fruit
Cascara Sagrada
Bark
Chamomile
Chickweed
Clivers
Comfrey
Counchgrass
Dandelion Root
Echinacea
Fennel
Globe Artichoke
Golden Seal
Licorice Root
Lobelia
Marsh mallow
Motherwort
Meadowsweet
Mullein
Peppermint
Raspberry Leaf*
Red Clover Tops
Rosehip
Rosemary
Slippery Elm
Squaw Vine
Thyme
Vervain
White Poplar
Yarrow
Yellow Dock

The previous table illustrates the plethora of remedies that have been recommended by various sources for the treatment of vaginal yeast infections. There is little information available on most of these substances.

Treating Yourself

Now that you're familiar with the four concepts involved in eliminating the pain and itching of candidal vaginitis, you can begin to examine specific yeast treatment options. The treatment sections are divided into three categories:

• home remedies,
• antifungal drug treatments, and
• nondrug antifungal treatments.

Home remedies are the least expensive, have had the fewest clinical trials, and often require the longest treatment time (typically fourteen days). They are readily available substances which have been shown to relieve the discomfort of yeast infections. Antifungal drug treatments are the most tested, most expensive options. They usually offer relief in three to seven days. Nondrug antifungals are substances whose primary action is antifungal; they are very effective, more costly than home remedies, but do not require a doctor's supervision. Nondrug antifungals typically afford relief in three to ten days.

Following these sections, information can be found on treatments for your sexual partner(s) as well as specific information for special situations, such as pregnancy, breast-feeding, and yeast infections in infants. Finally, this chapter concludes with some thoughts on yeast treatments of the future.

A plethora of remedies for yeast infections have

been recommended over the years by various sources. A partial list of these appears on page 148. Clinical trials have not been performed on the majority of these remedies; most nondrug antifungals and home remedies, in general, have received, at most, limited scientific scrutiny. In this country, pharmaceutical companies distribute the majority of the research funds. The result is endless studies on prescription drugs to the almost total exclusion of nondrug treatments. For instance, the sustained use of the powerful antifungal ketoconazole to treat candidal yeast infection can in some cases cause development of hepatitis in users. And, though high rates of subsequent yeast reinfection are well-known, too, the drug continues to be studied extensively. Yet there have been no studies on treatment with vinegar, an inexpensive remedy which has been used for decades by women around the world. While there are occasional studies on yogurt, one from South Africa and one from a Long Island, NY clinic, for instance, the overall lack of interest and funding in alternative treatment means that precise evaluation, exact dosages, the frequency and length of treatment are difficult to recommend. Until the scientific community decides to undertake evaluation of nonprescription treatments with the same extensive, systematic methods used to evaluate pharmaceuticals, women must continue to find out about alternative remedies through trial-and-error and word-of-mouth. Only when women are participants in determining research priorities will this situation change.

Much of the information presented here is anecdotal; it is a synthesis of recommendations from multiple respected sources, including medical journals, gynecologists, midwives, authoritative books on women's health, and women's groups. Many of the treatments have been shared woman-to-woman going back several generations. Experimenting on your own body will be your best guide to determine which remedies you find most effective.

All the treatments discussed are safe and may be practiced comfortably as long as you are not pregnant or breast-feeding (see the special cases section near the end of this chapter). However, in order for any of these remedies to work, you must have a correct diagnosis. As with every condition, before trying any of these self-help remedies, *make sure you are treating yeast*. Treating the wrong infection, or treating only one when you have multiple infections, may be harmful as it gives the infectious agent a chance to better establish itself in your body.

Remember, too, that Candida organisms cannot proliferate in the human body without heat and moisture. Before undertaking any treatment, try to minimize factors that promote candidal infection. Prevention tips can be found in chapter 6. Eliminating as many predisposing factors as possible will both reduce your need for treatment as well as lessen the severity of infections when they do strike. Chapter 2 reviews the common predisposing conditions. Knowing these yeast triggers will allow your treatment efforts to be undertaken as thoroughly as possible, allowing them to supplement the daily efforts you make toward prevention.

Finally, at the end of the home remedies section, there is a brief section with information on how to and how often to douche.

HOME REMEDIES

The remedies presented in this section have all been used by women to treat yeast infections. Each one is inexpensive and easily available. These compounds bring about change in the vaginal environment so that it becomes less hospitable to yeast organisms. Some have antifungal properties, but they are not considered primarily fungicidal. Compounds that are specifically antifungal are covered later in this chapter in the prescription and nonprescription treatment sections.

For the most part, the home remedies are not as strong as the formulations in the antifungal agents section. A key to using these remedies successfully is employing them at an early enough stage so that their strength will be sufficient for eradicating the condition. The more entrenched your infection is, the more difficult it will be to rid your body of it. Rather than waiting for a full-fledged infection, you might want to begin using the home remedies at the first sign of itching or immediately before your period if you are feeling particularly weak or tired that month.

The home remedies discussed in this section are: vinegar, yogurt, garlic, boric acid, homeopathic suppositories, Burows solution, aloe vera, and calendula cream. The first five are the most effective at providing symptomatic relief. The last three, used alone, can help ease the pain and irritation, but it is unlikely they could eliminate the symptoms of a yeast infection. They should be used in conjunction with the other remedies as a supporting way of reducing discomfort.

You can use the home remedies alone, in combination with other home remedies, or in combination with the antifungal drug or nondrug antifungal treatments. Using them in combination is your best bet for quick relief. In general, you will get the most relief if you use a remedy inside the vagina as well as one around the outer vaginal region (including around the anus). For instance, you may choose to use a boric acid suppository (to reach the inner vaginal region) while wearing aloe vera on a sanitary napkin (to help ease the redness and irritation of the outer area).

Home treatments should be taken seriously. Using vinegar douches (which create an environment less hospitable to yeast) while you consume brownies and doughnuts (which provide the sugars yeasts thrive on) may reduce the effectiveness of treatment. These treatments are meant to supplement the preventative changes made to your daily routine, as outlined in chapter 6.

These remedies are all for intravaginal use, and as such, are primarily aimed at relieving symptoms. Home treatments should only be used for up to a few weeks at a time. Do not practice any of these for prolonged periods of time. *If the symptoms do not abate within 14 days, you may be working with an incorrect diagnosis and you should see your health care provider.*

Vinegar

Women have been using acidic solutions, such as vinegar, in their vaginas since ancient Greece, and perhaps longer. Aristotle was one of the early medical men to suggest putting various solutions into the vagina in the quest for cleanliness and contraception. Because vinegar is so acidic, many people assume that the purpose of applying it is to lower the local pH. But yeasts, being very hardy organisms, can live quite contentedly in even a low pH environment. Vinegar is effective mostly because five different reactions begin in the vagina when the pH is lowered, all promoting good bacteria to the detriment of yeast.

The most important reaction when vaginal pH falls is the subsequent enhanced growth of healthy bacterial organisms, such as lactobacilli. An increase in lactobacilli production in turn hinders yeast growth in a variety of ways and restricts the growth of other harmful organisms by using up the very nutrients the yeasts need for their growth. Also, a healthy lactobacilli population sustains itself while maintaining the lower vaginal pH by producing lactic acid and hydrogen peroxide.

Second, while Candida can comfortably grow in an acidic environment, the ability of these yeast organisms to attach themselves to the vaginal cells falls as the pH declines. Free-floating rather than attached, they cannot attach themselves to the vaginal wall, and they cannot cause as high a degree of infection and discomfort.

Third, an acidic douche or preparation actually helps dry out the vagina. Candida organisms cannot survive without moisture, so the application of an acidic substance removing some of the moisture weakens the yeasts' ecosystem.

Fourth, the normal, healthy vagina is fairly acidic. In this state, the vaginal environment routinely employs a number of built-in defense mechanisms that daily protect you from disease-causing microorganisms, such as trichomonads. Maintaining a low pH helps to preserve overall vaginal health so you won't be susceptible to yeast infections in the first place.

Finally, in the process of acidifying the vagina, whether through a douche or preparation, you are actually diluting the microorganism population that lives there. Diluting the microorganism population can actually help wash away some of the yeasts, thus reducing their presence in your body.

Given these many beneficial results and the inexpensive cost and easy use of vinegar, it is no surprise that vinegar douches are a popular and effective treatment against mild yeast infections. Remember, however, that pure vinegar is a strong substance. Never apply it to your vagina without first diluting it. Preparing a mild solution is the first step. Commercial preparations or a too-strong one you prepare can trigger further discharge from damage to the vaginal cells, and leave you with an exacerbated condition. Four table-spoons of plain distilled white vinegar from the super-market in a pint of warm water is a fine douche solution. Do not use colored, seasoned, or flavored vinegar. Two douches a day should be sufficient.

There are many variations to a straight vinegar solution. Some women add some acidophilus powder or liquid to the douche mixture. Some use a solution of half warm water and half plain yogurt. Others use tepid herbal teas (raspberry leaf is a popular one) in place of plain water. Rather than using vinegar, a lemon douche achieves much the same result. A couple tablespoons of fresh juice to a pint of water makes a douche of appropriate strength. Lemon comes in handy especially if you find yourself on the road without douche equipment. Mix a little lemon juice in water and, with a clean finger, spread it around and inside your labia and vagina. An alternative to douching is to soak a tampon (O.B. brand works well) in a douche mixture and wear the tampon for a few hours.

While vinegar douches require a bit of effort, there is an effective, though costly, alternative. ACI-JEL, a prescription preparation from Ortho, is an exceptionally neat, convenient, and effective method of acid-ifying the vagina without the mess of douching. It is a bland, nonirritating, water-dispersible, buffered acid jelly for intravaginal use, with a pH of 4.0. The easiest way to think of it is thick vinegar in a toothpaste tube. ACI-JEL should be inserted twice daily into the vagina with an applicator; because of its thickness, the acid-ifying effects of ACI-JEL remain high for hours.

ACI-JEL works to restore and maintain normal vaginal acidity, but at approximately $35.00 for a three-ounce tube, it is outrageously expensive. Were it not for the expense, it would be handy to keep a tube around at all times. Unfortunately, if you are going to pay that kind of money for something, you are much better off buying an actual antifungal agent rather than thick vinegar. Nevertheless, ACI-JEL is a viable alternative to messy douches.

Yogurt

Yogurt, fermented milk with living bacterial microbes, has been used medicinally for centuries. Its claims to fame range from an effective treatment for intestinal infections to a technique for lowering blood cholesterol levels. It has been employed in the fight against heart disease, senility, and colon cancer. It is also a valuable tool in the battle against yeast vaginitis.

Douching with yogurt or inserting diluted yogurt into the vagina offers all the benefits of vinegar with one big added bonus: lactobacilli. Yogurt is not only acidic (plain yogurt has a pH of 4.5), it also is loaded with the lactobacilli organisms that play such a central role in restricting yeast growth and colonization. In fact, yogurt, just a tasty food to you, is a mixture of lactobacilli and nutrients not so much different from the mixture of the normal vaginal milieu.

Using yogurt to rid the body of yeast infections is probably the most popular home remedy among women. It is readily available and inexpensive and many women tell stories in which their success is almost mystically related to their particular method. One woman felt that goat yogurt was far superior to cow yogurt; another felt that the best technique was masturbating with yogurt to reap not only the benefits of the yogurt, but the healthy effects of the natural bodily secretions as well. Of course, eating yogurt will also increase the lactobacilli in your body and can help prevent yeast infections, though by itself it is not likely to rid your body of an established yeast infection.

There have only been two clinical studies of yogurt and yeast infections published in medical literature.

The *South African Medical Journal* reported a study in 1975 in which participants placed just under a teaspoon of commercial yogurt into their vaginas twice daily for one week, then twice weekly for two weeks. The results were quite encouraging: The application of yogurt significantly decreased the volume of discharge and the presence of vaginitis. The Long Island Jewish Medical Center in New York has been evaluating the results of research where women have been eating a cup of plain yogurt each day to reduce the incidence of chronic yeast infections. The preliminary findings indicate that regular ingestion of lactobacilli can be a powerful tool in helping the body ward off yeast infections.

Aside from eating yogurt, common methods of application include using a yogurt douche solution, "shooting" diluted yogurt into the vagina with a contraceptive-foam applicator, wearing yogurt on a sanitary pad, wearing a tampon soaked in yogurt, and using a clean finger to gently coat the vagina with yogurt. In any case, there is little point in using a brand of yogurt with few or no live lactobacilli cultures. Always use fresh, plain, unsweetened yogurt. Either buy a good brand at a health food store or pick one from the supermarket which is fresh and indicates that it contains live yogurt cultures. Adding an extra acidophilus supplement to the yogurt will turn the supermarket variety into a more potent source of lactobacilli.

A good douche solution is two-to-three heaping tablespoons of yogurt in a pint of warm water. For extra strength, add two tablespoons of plain vinegar to the mixture. Vinegar and yogurt can also be used in combination by first douching with vinegar, then using your finger to apply the yogurt to both the inside and outside of the vagina. You will want to wear a panty liner.

Garlic

Garlic is legendary in its healing properties and is used today almost universally. The beneficial properties of garlic have appeared in folklore and medical science from the beginnings of recorded history. The first written record of garlic was found around 5000 B.C. in Sanskrit writings. The Egyptians used garlic profusely; it is said that the builders of the pyramids would not work without their daily garlic rations. Several cloves were found in Tutankhamen's tomb, presumably to protect and preserve him. Greeks and Romans prescribed it for countless specific ailments as well as to build stamina and courage. The Romans considered it an aphrodisiac. Hippocrates advised using garlic for its natural healing qualities. In the Middle Ages, garlic was used to treat leprosy and to ward off evil spirits and vampires. At the turn of the century, it was widely used in the war against tuberculosis. The British purchased it by the ton and used it as an infection fighter in WWI, the Russians in WWII. Garlic has been prescribed over time as a cure or preventative for everything from acne to the plague.

While garlic may not be the ultimate elixir, its medical qualities should not be dismissed. It is one of the few abundant, nonproprietary medicines that has been scrutinized extensively by medical researchers. More than 1,000 scientific papers have been published on the various aspects of garlic. It is known to be an effective anticoagulant (blood thinner), used for years in China and Japan to treat high blood pressure. It also works well as an expectorant and decongestant and prevents the formation of plaque in atherosclerosis (which clogs up arteries) and reduces cholesterol levels. A survey of garlic and onion consumption in 20 countries showed that as the intake of these foods increases, the incidence of deaths from heart disease decreases. Garlic and onion may also play a role in keeping cholesterol levels low.

The Latin name for garlic is *Allium sativum*. It shares its family with lilies, leeks, onions, and scallions. It is a nutritionally superior food. An average clove contains only nine milligrams of sodium, thirty-one grams of protein (including all eight essential amino acids), calcium, iron, potassium, vitamins A, B1, B2, B3, C, and numerous minerals.

Folk medicine tells us that garlic rubbed on the feet will cure colds. It may not cure colds, but it might cure athlete's foot, because garlic is active against fungi. Not just an antifungal, garlic is also antiparasitic, anti-protozoan, and antiviral. Garlic aggressively inhibits fungal organisms and has been reported as more active against human ringworm (a fungal infection) than currently available drugs. It is said to cure cryptococcal meningitis (a frequently fatal fungal infection). Garlic is also considered to be an immune system booster, making garlic consumers better able to ward off disease.

Garlic cloves, placed right in the vagina, have been reported to be effective against yeast infections. This is a treatment option for pregnant women who do not want to douche or use drugs of any sort (check with your health practitioner before inserting anything in your vagina). Take a clove of garlic, remove the skin and nick the clove, wrap it in a cheesecloth (or leave it undressed) and insert it into the vagina. You can also pierce one or two garlic capsules (available in health food stores) and use them instead of fresh garlic cloves. Use one a day (before bedtime) or every twelve hours depending on the severity of the infection. (Note: The garlic is absorbed into the body through the mucous membranes, so don't be surprised if you find yourself tasting it the next day.)

Eat as much raw garlic (in salad dressings, casseroles, sauces, and other foods) as you can learn to enjoy. Your anti-Candida campaign should include daily intake of either fresh or deodorized garlic. Fresh garlic is best, but the capsules are an acceptable compromise. Nature's Way and Kyolic both produce odorless garlic capsules (available in health food stores); two capsules, morning and evening, after meals, will supplement your diet nicely.

Boric Acid

The notion of placing boric acid in the vagina brings horrific images to mind in many women because the most common association we have with it is as a pesticide, particularly effective against cockroaches. Most people don't realize that, in low concentrations, boric acid is nonirritating and suitable for many uses. Boric acid is commonly employed as an ingredient in eye drops, skin ointments, mouthwashes, skin powder, and hemorrhoidal suppositories.

Boric acid is an effective nondrug method of controlling yeast infections, one of the least expensive, most effective anticandida remedies known to woman. Treatment costs but pennies a day, and it is truly a sanity saver. Who wouldn't prefer to insert a neat, simple, odorless gelatin capsule rather than mess around with creams, applicators, douches, and soaking tampons? Boric acid can be used as a douche or in suppository form. Indeed, just about the hardest part of boric acid therapy (as a suppository) is finding the empty gelatin capsules to fill.

Boric acid alleviates symptoms as quickly as nystatin. It has been used widely throughout the southeastern United States with no untoward effects. In one study, boric acid users had significantly higher cure rates at both 10 and 30 days after treatment than nystatin users. The only side effect noted was a slight watery discharge during treatment. Of the women not

introduced in California where it was summarily taken off the market by the state department of Health and Human Services. Their issue was not the product, but the name, saying that the name encouraged women to diagnose and treat themselves—something they must not do. In response, the company withdrew the product from California, but sold it through the rest of the country. In the meantime, they reformulated and renamed the product for California, calling it Femicine. Femicine, also a package of 10 homeopathic suppositories, contains Pulsatilla, mercurius vivus, and sulfa (the latter two said to remove discharge). Satisfied with the product and the response in California, they then took Femicine nationwide. Two years later, after the FDA decided that women could safely diagnose and treat themselves, California let Yeast-Gard back in the state. Now both products are sold nationally and Femicine is the number-five selling feminine hygiene product sold in the U.S. mass market.

A new entry into the market seeking to share the wealth in homeopathic preparations is Yeast-X. Sold by the C. B. Fleet Company (makers of enemas, Summer's Eve douches, and Norforms), a box of twelve suppositories with applicator sells for $7.00. Yeast-X suppositories contain only Pulsatilla.

As with most suppositories, these products might cause a slight discharge. A panty liner is suggested to protect clothing and provide maximum comfort.

The market success of Yeast-Gard is an indicator of how eager women are to have affordable symptomatic relief. A ten-day supply of Yeast-Gard is almost half the price of a seven-day tube of Gyne-Lotrimin or Monistat 7.

Burows Solution

Wet dressings or soaks with Burows solution are another suggested way to combine vulvar hygiene and healing. You can use this astringent solution, mainly aluminum acetate, as a wet dressing for relief of many inflammatory conditions of the skin; it is even used against athlete's foot, a fungal infection. It helps damaged areas to clean, dry, and heal, and provides immediate soothing relief for ulcerations or open sores.

The easiest way to use Burows solution is to buy the Domeboro powder (available at most drugstores without prescription) and prepare it according to the directions on the packet. Make a wet compress by applying the solution to gauze or a sanitary pad. It can be prepared lukewarm or cold. Some women find it extra soothing if they refrigerate the solution and apply the cooled liquid. Leave the wet compress in place for half an hour, adding more solution if necessary to keep the compress wet. Use the compresses two to three times a day; after each treatment dry your vaginal area.

No side effects should be expected. If you find it uncomfortable for any reason, stop and try a different remedy.

Aloe Vera

The aloe plant has been used as a medicinal for millennia. In 333 B.C., Alexander the Great was told of the plant and sent a commission to the island of Socotra to bring him a sample. Aloes have been used in the treatment of chronic constipation, amenorrhea (missed periods), and as an analgesic and healer for burns, scrapes, sunburn, and insect bites. It is commonly used to treat burn victims because of its soothing and healing qualities. Its use is not limited to victims burned by fire; it is also used in the treatment of radiation burns on patients undergoing X-ray treatment for cancer and related diseases. Aloe has been found, in fact, to be a most effective treatment for all minor radiation burns.

Aloe vera can also be used for vaginal care. It has a pH almost identical to that of a healthy vagina while its soothing and healing qualities provide quick, fast relief of vaginal itching, redness, and minor pain.

The easiest form to work with is an aloe vera gel; Aloe Products sells a 16 ounce bottle of gel for approximately $5.00. It can be used as a douche (mix one-third cup to a pint of warm water) or inserted directly into the vagina (apply two teaspoonfuls into the vagina). The solution can be applied as one-to-two tablespoons on a sanitary pad, too.

Calendula Cream

The extract of the calendula flower (a flower similar to the marigold) has been recognized for decades for its healing qualities. Used widely in Europe, formulas prepared with calendula help heal and soothe rough, chapped skin, cuts, burns, and inflammations. In 1955 a patent was issued in Austria for the use of extracts of marigold flowers as an emollient in the treatment of burns in humans. It is considered a natural antiseptic by homeopaths. Calendula formulations have been used to soothe watery irritated eyes, to provide relief for bronchial sufferers, and to lower blood pressure.

Calendula creams or gels are available at health food stores and homeopathic pharmacies. They have an acidity level very similar to that of a healthy vagina. Try Marigold Ointment (NatureWorks, 1.75 ounces for $5.65) or Calendula Cream from Hyland Homeopathics (1-ounce tube for $3.29). Creams and gels can be applied liberally to the outer vagina, several times a

HOME REMEDY PREPARATIONS
FOR SYMPTOMATIC RELIEF

Use Inside Vagina (intravaginal)	*Use Outside Vagina* (extravaginal)
Vinegar douche	
Vinegar-soaked tampon	
Lemon douche	
Yogurt*	Yogurt
Yogurt douche	
Yogurt-soaked tampon	
Acidophilus capsules*	
Acidophilus douche	
Boric acid douche	Boric acid ointment
Boric acid suppositories	
Homeopathic suppositories	
Garlic cloves*	
Garlic capsules*	
Aloe vera	Aloe vera
Aloe vera douche	
	Burows solution
	Calendula cream

*These items also have medicinal value when eaten.

day. Gels can also be soaked into a sanitary pad (one to three tablespoons) and worn for several hours.

To increase effectiveness and speed up the relief from irritation, home remedies should include treatment inside the vagina as well as a cream or ointment around the outer vaginal tissues, the vaginal lips, and the anal region. Any of the home remedies can be used alone, in combination with other home remedies, or in combination with any of the antifungal drug or nondrug treatments.

On page 168 is a chart of the various home remedies you can use both intra- and extravaginally. Use a treatment from each side of the chart, so that you are able to cover the whole genital region. You can try a variety of remedies to see which ones provide you the most effective symptomatic relief.

Douching

The vagina is an amazing ecosystem which keeps itself clean and healthy while providing just the right environment for sperm to reach their destination. It has its own regular internal cleansing process, so normally there is no reason to douche, or rinse out the vagina, other than as part of a prevention or treatment program. There are times, however, when a little intervention can go a long way. Sometimes, a good rinsing gives the body a boost in ridding itself of undesirable organisms, allows you to introduce desired organisms, and lets you alter the pH of the vagina.

Douching should not be done routinely. The repeated drying effect of multiple douches may actually increase vaginal discharge. While it is still too early to be considered conclusive, two recent studies suggest that women who douche frequently have a higher risk of contracting pelvic inflammatory disease (PID) and cervical cancer. Although douching is unnecessary for healthy women, women with yeast vaginitis may find douching a helpful tool for preventing or fending off an infection, especially at times of increased susceptibility such as around menstruation. Always douche with a gentle, nonscented solution; commercial or harsh preparations often produce a further discharge by damaging the vaginal epithelial cells, or even producing allergic reactions.

Douche bags are available in most drugstores. There are two varieties, the bag-and-hose kind and the hand-held kind, each sells for $7 to $11. The former allows you to reach deeper in the vaginal cavity with more pressure, the latter is smaller and easier to assemble and carry. Always douche gently, taking care not to squeeze the bag hard. Too much pressure can force air or fluid up into the uterus, and even into the abdominal cavity. It is best to douche with a lukewarm solution. When using the bag-and-hose method, hang or hold the bag about one or two feet above your hips, about at the top of the bathtub when you're sitting in it. Wait until the air is out of the tubing and the solution is running before putting the nozzle into your vagina. Pregnant women should check with their health practitioners before douching and, when douching, insert the nozzle only slightly into the vagina, applying very gentle pressure.

The suggested regime for douching varies with its purpose. For prevention or mild infections, douche once or twice daily for three to five days; for severe infections, douche twice daily for the first five to seven days, then once daily for the next five to seven days. *If the infection has not cleared within two weeks, consult your primary care provider.* Be sure to make an appointment at least two days after your last douche so that the vaginal milieu can be examined in an unaltered state. You should never douche within two days of a gynecological exam.

Some Rules for Douching:

• The container, tube, and irrigation nozzle should be kept very clean and dried thoroughly before storage. Unclean douche equipment can provide a home for yeast organisms. Wash the equipment with hot water and soap or a good antiseptic solution. You might also try using a mild vinegar solution to wash it. Sun drying will also help destroy resident yeast organisms.

• The optimal position for douching is lying in a bathtub with your legs spread apart. A folded towel placed under your rear end will make this position more comfortable (and warmer) while it helps lift your pelvic region so the douche fluids can penetrate deeply.

• Using a gentle rotating motion, insert the nozzle into your vagina. Once you encounter pressure, stop. The nozzle will generally go in about two to four inches.

• Allow the solution to flow in slowly and try to hold the liquids inside you as long as possible. Some women use their fingers to hold the vaginal lips closed while a little pressure builds up to help the solution coat the internal surfaces.

Two alternatives to douching are to soak a natural sea sponge (generally sold as menstrual sponges in health food stores) in your douching solution and wear it in your vagina or soak a tampon (O.B. brand works well) in the solution and insert it. Wear either the sponge or tampon for several hours or overnight. These should be changed regularly and, in the case of the sponge, cleaned and dried thoroughly. Nothing (a sea sponge, tampon, or diaphragm for example) should be left in the vagina for more than eight to ten hours; that is how toxic shock syndrome occurs.

ANTIFUNGAL DRUG TREATMENTS

The choice of drug therapies offered to physicians for treating vaginal candidiasis is confusingly large. There are over a dozen specific prescription antifungal medications available in formulations that include oral tablets, oral powders, oral liquids, topical powders, genital creams, genital ointments, vaginal suppositories, and coated tampons. There are a handful of drug remedies available over-the-counter that until recently had been sold only as prescription. From this vast array of antifungal drugs, a doctor may choose any treatment regime from a one-time suppository to a long-term combined regime of creams and oral tablets. The most common treatments are creams and suppositories prescribed for a three- to seven-day period.

These anticandida drugs all belong chemically to one of two groups: the polyene group and the imidazole derivative group. Within the polyene group, nystatin is the most commonly used medication. Within the imidazole derivative group, there are five common medications: miconazole, clotrimazole, butoconazole, terconazole, and ketoconazole. This section focuses on the various treatment options involved in intravaginal treatment (suppositories, creams, ointments, and tablets). You can find the pros and cons of oral treatment earlier in this chapter in the section "Reduce the Yeast Population of the Gastrointestinal Tract."

While there are various modes of topical application from which to choose, the choice appears to have little effect on the outcome of treatment. The primary cure rates between both groups of drugs don't vary much either, with disappearance of symptoms for a primary cure in 80–90 percent of cases. Creams and ointments have a primary cure rate around 88 percent, tablets and suppositories around 85 percent.

Many women comment that they feel the creams work better than the suppositories. This may be due to the fact that a cream covers more surface area than a suppository and may therefore reach (and destroy) more potential yeast organisms. Additionally, creams offer three important bonuses over a suppository. With one prescription, a cream provides a medication useful on the vulva and vagina, and around the anus as a preventative. The same medication can also be used by your sex partner. The main complaint about creams is the need to wash the applicators after each use. If you do not have a strong preference of fluid versus solid application, ask for a cream.

The recommended duration of topical treatment ranges from one to thirty days depending on the specific drug and delivery form. Generally speaking, the stronger the formulation, the shorter the treatment; for instance, clotrimazole tablets for one-time use are 500 mg, while the tablets for seven-day use are 100 mg. Choosing between a stronger short-use treatment and a milder longer-use regime is not an especially crucial decision. All the formulations are safe and have been demonstrated to be at least 80 percent effective in providing symptomatic relief against candida vaginitis when used according to the manufacturers' directions. *Symptomatic relief, however, does not guarantee eradication of the disease.*

All of the formulations were sold as prescription drugs until 1991. A few years earlier, the makers of Gyne-Lotrimin (clotrimazole) and Monistat (nystatin) applied for and were granted a reclassification of their products to over-the-counter (OTC) status. The OTC formulations are identical to the ones sold as prescription. This has created a situation that is good for the consumer, but is a bit bizarre as the drugs in the same strength are available both as prescriptions and as drugstore shelf items under different names. The story of how the reclassification came about is told in Appendix D.

Interestingly, the same drugs have also been available in the same strength for over a decade as topical creams for athlete's foot. These could easily be used instead of the vaginal preparations but there is no price advantage and you don't get an applicator with your purchase. When traveling overseas, an athlete's foot preparation may be the easiest answer to a sudden case of yeast vaginitis or diaper rash.

The following agents are available in the United States in intravaginal and/or oral formulations for use against yeast infections.

Developed almost 40 years ago, nystatin has been around the longest. The imidazoles are more recent developments. Miconazole first became available as a cream for vulvovaginal candidiasis in 1974, terconazole in 1988. The newer drugs have not been shown to be

ANTIFUNGAL DRUG TREATMENTS

	Generic Name	Proprietary Name	Delivery Vehicle
Polyene antibiotics	Nystatin	Nystatin	Oral/Vaginal
	Nystatin	Nilstat	Oral/Vaginal
	Nystatin	Nystex	Oral/Vaginal
	Nystatin	Mycostatin	Vaginal
Imidazole derivatives	Clotrimazole	Mycelex	Vaginal
	Clotrimazole	Gyne-Lotrimin*	Vaginal
	Miconazole	Monistat*	Vaginal
	Butoconazole	Femstat	Vaginal
	Terconazole	Terazol	Vaginal
	Ketoconazole	Nizoral	Oral/Vaginal

*Available as over-the-counter.

significantly more or less effective than the standard bearer, nystatin.

For the treatment of vaginal candidal infections, the most commonly used drugs, their trade names, and the cost for one course of treatment (as of mid-1991 in the New York metropolitan area) are listed on pages 176–77.

Johnson and Johnson has had a virtual lock on the market for prescription remedies. With their Monistat and Terazol products, Johnson and Johnson, owners of Ortho Pharmaceuticals, control over 80 percent of the market. In 1990, its last year as a prescription drug, Monistat was the top-selling vaginal antifungal preparation, holding 55 percent of the market and generating $120 million in annual sales. Monistat 7 has been prescribed 70,000,000 times since it was introduced in 1977. Terazol, a cream containing terconazole, held 28 percent of the market in 1990. Now that the number of vaginal yeast preparations has increased and Gyne-Lotrimin and Monistat 7 are over-the-counter, there will be shifts in the market, although loosening Johnson and Johnson's hold remains a challenge.

Nystatin

Nystatin is an antifungal antibiotic that kills yeast organisms by disrupting their cell membranes. It is deadly against a wide variety of yeasts while leaving bacteria unharmed. It was the first fast-acting, well-tolerated pharmaceutical for the treatment of infections caused by Candida yeasts. It is a contact fungicide, killing the fungi only by coming into direct contact with them.

One of nystatin's greatest strengths and weaknesses is that it is poorly absorbed into the bloodstream. When taken orally, the majority of the dose goes into the stomach, passes on to the intestines, then con-

COMPARATIVE COSTS OF ANTIFUNGAL DRUGS

Product Name	Drug Name	Delivery Vehicle	Cost
Mycostatin	Nystatin	7 day; 15 100,000 U vaginal tablets	$17.00
Generic	Nystatin (pure powder in capsules)	7 day; 15 100,000 U capsules	$ 8.60
Generic	Nystatin (pure powder)*	25 day; 10 grams of powder (1 tsp = 5,000,000 U)	$20.85
Femstat	Butoconazole	3 day; 2% cream; 28 grams	$21.70
Femstat	Butoconazole	3 day; 2% cream; filled disposable applicators	$22.95
Monistat**	Miconazole	7 day; 2% cream; 1.59 ounces	$22.49
Monistat	Miconazole	3 day; 200 mg vaginal suppositories	$27.25
Monistat**	Miconazole	7 day; 100 mg vaginal suppositories	$22.49
Monistat***	Miconazole	3/7 day; 3 day suppositories and small tube of cream	$29.25

Gyne-Lotrimin**	Clotrimazole	7 day; 1% cream; 1.5 ounces
Gyne-Lotrimin**	Clotrimazole	7 day; 100 mg vaginal suppositories
Mycelex	Clotrimazole	1 day; 500 mg vaginal tablet
Mycelex	Clotrimazole	7 day; 100 mg vaginal tablet
Mycelex	Clotrimazole	7 day; 100 mg vaginal tablets
Mycelex***	Clotrimazole	7 day; 1% cream; 45 grams
Mycelex***	Clotrimazole	1/7 day; 1 500 mg tablet and small tube of cream
Terazole	Terconazole	7 day; 0.4% cream

			$22.49
			$22.49
			$15.75
			$19.30
			$18.40
			$19.15
			$19.10

*It may be difficult to purchase quantities less than 10 grams.

**Sold as over-the-counter drugs.

***Although sold for one course of treatment, these combination packages contain suppositories for use inside the vagina and a small tube of topical cream for use outside the vagina.

tinues on to the bowel. The fact that it does not get absorbed systemically accounts for its effectiveness in clearing yeast infections, especially those of the lower intestines and the bowel.

Nystatin was discovered in 1949, isolated from an actinomycete, a funguslike bacteria, found in the pasture of a dairy farm in Fouquier County, Virginia. The organism produced two antifungal antibiotics. One was identified as "actidione," the other was named "nystatin" (after the New York State laboratory where the researchers worked). It has proved safe throughout decades of widespread use. Other fungicidal drugs have been around longer, but their use is limited by their toxicity. Even though newer antifungals have become available, nystatin continues to be a mainstay of candidiasis therapy.

Nystatin is commonly sold under the brand name Mycostatin, but it is also available under other brand names and as a generic. It is used in liquid form to treat yeast growth in the mouth (oral thrush); as oral tablets, powder, and pastilles for yeast infection of the intestinal tract; as ointments, powders, creams, and aerosols for infections of the skin and nails (including diaper rash). As a cream, ointment, and suppository, it is very effective against vaginal candidiasis. Additionally, as a generic drug, it is available in pure powder form. The powder is less expensive and slightly more effective than the prepared forms, but may be harder to find (see page 146 for instructions to purchase it by mail). The powder can be taken orally or enclosed in gelatin capsules and used as suppositories. Note: The powder form should be refrigerated; all other forms are stable at room temperature.

Nystatin is considered virtually nontoxic. Patients of all ages and strengths, from debilitated infants to AIDS victims, generally accept the drug without significant side effects. Prolonged treatment is considered safe; neither primary resistance nor the development of resistant strains of fungi have been problems in people undergoing prolonged nystatin therapy. Additionally, intravaginal use of nystatin is considered safe during pregnancy. Its safety during breast-feeding has not been established. Nystatin formulations should be used once or twice daily until three days after symptoms have disappeared. Do not discontinue use during menstruation.

The Imidazoles

In the United States, four major topical forms of imidazoles are used against vaginal candidiasis: butoconazole, clotrimazole, miconazole, and terconazole. In addition, ketoconazole is also a member of this drug class, but has not been approved for vaginal candidiasis due to its toxicity. The four approved, commonly used topical imidazoles will be discussed here. Separate information on ketoconazole is contained in the next section.

The imidazoles are synthetic broad-spectrum antifungal agents. They are considered safe and effective when used topically against vaginal candidiases. They destroy yeast organisms while leaving unaffected the beneficial bacteria of the vaginal tract. There have been no reports of primary resistance to the imidazoles, nor of the emergence of resistant strains of Candida or other fungi during treatment. Used intravaginally, they are poorly absorbed into the bloodstream.

As with most topical agents, side effects with the imidazoles are quite rare. In a low percentage of cases, women find they have a hypersensitivity to these imidazoles. Stop using the medication and see your health care giver if you experience local irritation, mild burning, skin rash, and/or itching. Lower abdominal pain, cramps, bloating, slight urinary frequency, and irritation in the sexual partner have been reported, but the nature of vaginitis makes it hard to tell whether these events are drug related or disease related.

The choice of which approved topical imidazole treatment to use is not crucial. All the ones tested and approved for yeast vaginitis, when used correctly, are essentially interchangeable. If you have a preference, let your care giver know. Cost may be an important consideration to some, delivery method may be more important to others. Still others consider length of treatment. The chart on pages 176–77 showing type of application, length of treatment, and cost may help you determine which drug antifungal you prefer. One consideration is that, statistically speaking, the shorter the course of therapy, the more likely people are to complete the prescription.

When choosing which imidazole to use, there are several considerations. The base ingredient in the suppository formulation may interact with certain latex products, like diaphragms or condoms. If you plan on being sexually active during treatment, a cream is therefore preferable to suppositories. You should continue to use the medications through your menstrual cycle if those days are part of your program, but you can't use tampons since they may absorb the medication instead of your body.

Clotrimazole is the only imidazole available in a single-day dose. Suppositories are generally used in the single treatment and three-day treatments, while creams are designed for six- to seven-day regimes (butoconazole is the only cream available in a three-day formulation). Creams may not offer the shortest course of treatment, but a cream does provide, in one tube, medication for the vagina, the vulva, the anus, and the partner.

The best bet is a three- to seven-day treatment. One-shot treatments may not be as effective (in which case, you've just thrown away your money), while length of treatment alone (superlong-term, for example) does not guarantee success. For instance, the package insert for one of the clotrimazole creams states that there is a statistically improved benefit when used for a full 14 days. In a double-blind study comparing the 7-day and the 14-day regimens, however, no statistical difference at all was found in cure rates.

As a general rule, creams are considered safer than suppositories for pregnant women. Pregnant women also require up to twice the treatment regime as their nonpregnant counterparts, typically a seven-day program at a minimum. (See the special cases section of this chapter for more information on treatments during pregnancy.) During pregnancy, clotrimazole and miconazole are considered the safest of the imidazole derivatives, although no adequate and well-controlled studies have been conducted with these during the first trimester. Use of these products in the second and third trimesters has not been associated with any ill effects. Butoconazole and terconazole are not recommended for pregnant women, and should only be used in the second and third trimesters, if at all. The effect of imidazoles on breast milk has also not been extensively studied; all imidazole preparations should be used with caution by nursing mothers. Nursing mothers, as a rule, should try home remedies first if they get yeast infections. The safety and effectiveness of the imidazoles for children has not been established.

The main thing to keep in mind is that the topical imidazoles (and nystatin for that matter) are effective in alleviating symptoms though they are significantly more expensive than home remedies. All of these therapies boast quite satisfactory initial cure rates. Unfortunately, they also all claim significant recurrence rates as well. While some women may say a permanent farewell to their infections after a single course of an antifungal drug treatment, others will find the relief short-lived since recurrence is the hallmark of this disease. In all cases, you should discontinue their use two-to-three days after your symptoms have cleared up and focus your efforts on the more long-term strategy to overcome your predisposition to yeast infections.

If your symptoms persist, you may have been incorrectly diagnosed and should visit your health care provider.

Ketoconazole

Ketoconazole is a synthetic broad-spectrum antifungal agent. It was introduced into the U.S. market a few years ago in the form of oral tablets, distributed by Janssen Pharmaceutical and sold under the brand name Nizoral. Nizoral has recently been made available as a cream for topical use. Neither the tablets nor the cream have been approved for routine use in the treatment of vaginal candidiasis, but some doctors do use them and clinical trials for this purpose have been conducted. (Be sure to have your liver enzymes tested regularly for hepatoxicity if you do use oral ketoconazole.)

Ketoconazole is a powerful antifungal, most commonly used for *tinea corporis*, a stubborn fungal infection of the finger- and toenails. It can also be effective against obstinate athlete's foot and ringworm. For cases of deep-rooted fungal infections, it is more effective than nystatin.

Besides the fact that it has not been approved for vaginal candidiases treatment, there are some significant reasons to stay far away from ketoconazole. In study after study, it has been found to offer no real improvement in efficacy over other available treatments nor has it proved significantly better in preventing recurrences.

It would appear that oral ketoconazole would be a viable long-term solution (very few women had infections while they were taking the pills), except that its side effects are very serious. They include: severe nausea, severe itching, vomiting, abdominal pain, headaches, dizziness, allergies, skin rashes and, most importantly, the risk of liver damage. Worse, the liver damage is independent of dose, so taking a small dose is not necessarily safer. The seriousness of developing hepatitis is great enough that anyone taking ketoconazole must undergo careful (and costly) monitoring of the liver enzymes throughout the course of treatment and after. Putting yourself at risk of liver damage (two out of forty-five women experienced reversible hepatitis in one study) seems totally unnecessary for a cure that is not significantly better than other available antifungals with relatively minor side effects. Additionally, some drug interactions have been reported with ketoconazole usage.

Side effects of the cream include severe irritation, itching, stinging, and allergic reactions. Additionally, the cream contains sulfites, which may cause allergic reactions in sensitive individuals, especially asthmatics.

Within our current body of knowledge, there is no reason to use this drug for treating vaginal yeast infections.

NONDRUG ANTIFUNGAL AGENTS

The choice between drug and nondrug treatments is one of personal preference. Nondrug antifungal medications can be used by themselves or in conjunction with drug formulations. All the nondrug antifungals are proven safe and boast effectiveness rates comparable to the antifungal drug preparations discussed here.

What is the difference between a nondrug antifungal and a home remedy? Both are effective. The home remedies work for a variety of reasons, by supplementing bacteria or drying the vagina, for example, but are not primarily antifungal in nature. The home remedies can be found in almost any drugstore or supermarket. The nondrug antifungals are specific agents whose primary mode of action is the destruction of yeast organisms. They should be easily obtainable in the larger drugstores and health food stores.

After years of struggling with yeast infections, and following "doctor's orders," many women have elected to bypass the medical establishment altogether and stick with nondrug treatments. The next section describes three nondrug antifungals: caprylic acid (used with sorbic acid), povidone-iodine, and gentian violet. The main advantages and disadvantages of each are discussed below.

One big advantage to these nondrug antifungals is that you don't need a doctor's permission to purchase and use them (or to get refills). This means you may be able to start treatment sooner, with less disruption to your daily schedule. The disadvantage is that without seeing a doctor, you may be misdiagnosing your condition, treating a problem other than the one you actually have with all the potential health consequences that postponing the correct treatment entails.

Another advantage is that many of the nonprescription medications have been used for years and have passed the test of time. They are not only known among women as things that work, but they have all passed Food and Drug Administration testing for safety and effectiveness. The disadvantage is that, being outside the major medical model, these treatments have not been investigated as systematically and with the same rigor as prescription drugs.

Finally, nondrug antifungals usually cost less than the antifungal drug medications; home remedies cost even less. The money you can save by treating yourself can easily add up to hundreds of dollars—not including the cost of the medical visit(s) you need in order to get a prescription! Of course, if you do have good insurance coverage, the expense of prescription drugs may be fully or substantially reimbursable, whereas health insurance companies will rarely pay for nonprescription medications, even if taken at the direction of a physician.

One disadvantage to nondrug treatments is that they generally need to be used for longer periods of time than antifungal drug treatments. One to seven days of use are the norm in the antifungal drug world, while seven to fourteen days is more common with these preparations. This is not because the medications are less effective. Indeed, the cure rates seem to be similar. Rather, nondrug antifungals appear to act differently on the yeast and simply need to be used longer to achieve the same result.

Finally, another disadvantage to nondrug treatments is that they are consistently more messy to use than the neatly packaged drug formulations. Some women are quite adept at preparing home treatments, but for most people, preparing douche mixtures, soaking tampons, and working with many of these substances is not their first choice for ways to spend free time. Drug formulations come in concisely measured quantities wrapped in neat little packages with disposable applicators.

All the treatments suggested for candidiasis in this book are available, effective, and safe, if used correctly. The selection of which are best for you depends on a number of factors and are not the same for everyone.

Caprylic Acid

> When combined with other natural antifungal substances, such as garlic and yogurt, caprylic acid may achieve a broader spectrum of antiyeast activity than can many prescription drugs now used against established yeast infections.
>
> —Drs. Trowbridge and Walker, *The Yeast Syndrome*

Caprylic acid is short-chain fatty acid that is present in coconut oil. Fatty acids have long been known for their antifungal activity; of all the fatty acids, caprylic acid is effective against all Candida species. Taken orally (caprylic acid is only available for oral use), it can help restore and maintain a healthy balance of yeast, bacteria, and other microorganisms throughout the gastrointestinal region. Caprylic acid is not a new discovery; its prompt and effective response against yeast organisms has been documented since the 1940s.

Like nystatin, caprylic acid is a contact fungicide that is not absorbed by the body. Since stomach acids can break it down, reducing its effectiveness before it gets to the yeast-rich large and small intestines, most commercially available caprylic acid preparations are coated so that they pass through the stomach to the lower intestinal tract. For this reason, they should be swallowed whole. Since you want the antifungal activity to continue over a period of time, a timed-release tablet is the most effective.

Caprylic acid is safe and tasteless. Like nystatin, it is not absorbed into the bloodstream, so toxicity is not an issue. No adverse side effects have been observed when taken at recommended dosage levels, though very large doses can cause gastrointestinal irritation and produce diarrhea, nausea, and vomiting. Caprylic acid does have a high fiber content, and may act as a mild laxative. All of the information presented here does not apply to pregnant or breast-feeding women, or children up to 12, groups for whom there have been no extensive studies.

Other than the laxative response, the only repercussion you may experience when taking caprylic acid is what is known as the Herxheimer effect. This refers to fatigue and flulike symptoms that may occur during the first two to five days of use, and which will stop completely by the end of the first week. Just as with nystatin use, the Herxheimer effect is thought to result from large numbers of yeast suddenly dying off inside your gastrointestinal tract and releasing toxins. This reaction is not considered a side effect, rather, it is a positive indication that the antifungal is working. Because of the possibility of a Herxheimer reaction, it is best to start on half the regular dosage and work up to a full dosage over a seven- to ten-day period. If the reaction is too unpleasant, cut the dosage way back and work up gradually or try switching brands.

There are numerous commercially available caprylic acid products. Caprystatin by Ecological Formulas was the first formulation on the market, introduced in 1984. Since Caprystatin hit the stores, numerous other products have become available, some with caprylic acid only, others combining caprylic acid with other antifungal agents and/or nutritional supplements. Tablets usually contain 100 mg of caprylic acid. The usual dosage is two tablets, two times daily for one month, followed by two months at half dosage. If you experience any bloating, headaches, or fatigue, reduce the dosage or change brands. Different companies bond the caprylic acid to different bases so some brands may work better for your body. A list of some of the caprylic acid formulations appears on page 147. Caprylic acid can also be an effective preventative of yeast infections when taking antibiotics (see "Guide to Taking Antibiotics" in chapter 6).

Unlike oral caprylic acid treatment, sorbic acid, another fatty acid with antifungal properties, can be used directly in the vagina. It can be used as a douche or applied by saturating a tampon with the solution and wearing it for two hours, twice a day. Ecological Formulas' product, Orithrush Vaginal Douche Concentrate ($14.95 for 8 ounces), provides women with an effective nonprescription formulation for local application to complement oral use. Like all the vaginal treatments, these should not be used daily, but only for short periods (up to 14 days) when symptomatic relief is required.

Povidone-Iodine

Povidone-iodine is a long-standing treatment for vaginal yeast infections. In fact, it is effective against yeast, trichomonads, combined yeast and trich infections, as well as some cases of nonspecific vaginitis. It is a treatment which has been in use for many years and today is available in both prescription and nonprescription preparations.

Povidone-iodine is a broad-spectrum antiseptic that can be purchased as a douche, gel, or suppository. Unlike antifungals, antiseptics kill both bacteria and yeast, therefore you should only use povidone-iodine as part of a treatment program, not routinely.

When used correctly, povidone-iodine boasts some of the most successful short- and long-term cure rates of any of the medications. Rates as high as 100 percent for yeast infections, 98 percent for trichomonal infections, 93 percent for mixed trich-yeast infections, and 70 percent for women with nonspecific vaginitis have been reported. Additionally, relapse rates three months after therapy are reported to be as low as 2.8 percent.

Povidone-iodine, however, is not without side effects: A small percentage of women will experience vulvar itching and/or minor discomfort. Severe swelling, vulvar inflammation, and painful stinging can also occur. An offensive odor may also arise from the treatment. Be sure to wear a panty liner during treatment, because your discharge may be yellowish-brown. Don't worry, this is water-soluble and will come out with normal laundering. If the side effects are manageable, grin and bear it—they rarely last more than three days. If they are too unpleasant, stop the povidone-iodine and try another approach.

Povidone-iodine is available in a variety of forms. The Women's Health Institute sells a povidone-iodine douche concentrate. An 8-ounce bottle sells for $9.15 and makes 16 douches. Purdue Frederick Co. also sells an 8-ounce bottle of concentrate that makes 16 douches for $11.89. Disposable premade douches are available in most drugstores. Betadine and Summer's Eve disposable douches contain povidone-iodine. A single douche costs around $2.50, the twin packs range from $3.50 to $5.00. Medicated suppositories, produced by Bard Pharmaceuticals, in packages of seven (with an applicator) sell for $12.29. A 3-ounce tube of Betadine vaginal gel is also available (comes with an applicator) at a cost of $18.69. Whichever of these you choose, they should be used for a minimum of 14 days. Studies have shown that shorter treatment times result in significantly higher failure rates. For women with stubborn cases and those taking oral contraceptives, a 28-day course of treatment has demonstrated quite impressive results. This may be a viable option for those who feel they are close to eradicating the problem, but have not quite succeeded.

Women who are pregnant, planning on becoming pregnant soon, or nursing should not use povidone-iodine. Also, allergies to it are not uncommon. Women who have iodine-sensitivity and/or allergies to seafood may find they are better off using one of the many other antiyeast treatments rather than risking any reaction to the povidone-iodine.

Gentian Violet

Gentian violet is another long-used treatment for thrush. It is commonly used the world over for oral thrush in children, as a topical preparation for fungal infections of the skin, and as a routine remedy for burns.

Gentian violet is a dye. It is extremely messy to use, staining everything it comes into contact with, including your skin, a deep blue. Gentian violet has fallen into disuse, not because it doesn't work (it certainly does), but simply because it stains so easily. Gentian violet concentrate can be found at most drugstores, but it is not always easy to locate. Ask the pharmacist for assistance if you run into difficulty. It is a rich deep purple liquid with a slight odor of alcohol.

Gentian violet can be used intravaginally in a variety of ways. Most commonly, it is used either as a douche or as a suppository (soaked into a tampon). Dilute one half a teaspoon of concentrate into eight ounces of water and use twice daily. One bottle containing 30 cc of gentian violet sells for $2.95. The main side effect is staining. Be sure to wear a sanitary napkin and old underwear.

Gentian violet is also available as a prescription, although the cost would send any sane person to find a cheaper alternative. Gentian violet tampons, under the brand name Genepax (Key Pharmaceuticals), are sold for use against vaginal yeast infections. Twelve tampons sell for $28.00. The recommended treatment is to wear one or two tampons a day, leaving them in place for three to four hours at a time, for 12 days. If irritation, swelling, or pain develop, discontinue use.

TREATMENT AND PREVENTION FOR THE PARTNER

> There is an element of sexual transmissibility in candidiasis. Cases in males have increased by about 100 percent and female cases by about 14 percent between 1971 and 1975. The ratio of male to female cases has changed from nearly one to eight in 1971 to about one to five in 1975.
>
> —Drs. Morton and Rashid,
> *Proceedings of the Royal Society of Medicine*

Yeast infections strike women regardless of how sexually active they are. Certainly, your infections are not necessarily related to your sex life. However, sexual transmission can be a factor contributing to your condition, for researchers estimate that yeast infections are sexually acquired in approximately 39 percent of women's episodes and 29 percent of heterosexual men's episodes. Sexual transmission is not normally the primary source of yeast problems (since an altered physiological state or debility must occur first), but for some women such contact may trigger or exacerbate chronic infections.

Doctors often dismiss any role the partner may play in instigating infections, though we have known for over a hundred year that infected nipples, unsterilized pacifiers, bottles, and diapers have been implicated in transmitting infantile thrush. While sexual transmissibility is unlikely to be the only factor in recurrent vulvovaginal candidiases, the vagina-penis-vagina cycle of transmission may account for reinfection in women, especially those struggling with chronic infection. If you are having trouble with recurring infections and feel there may be a correlation between sexual activity and outbreaks, you should see that your partner gets treated, something that is neither difficult nor harmful and may eliminate an important source of reinfection. (Here we talk about male partners; women with female partners will find information at the end of this section as well as in chapter 2.)

If you have yeast infections, there is a high probability that your partner is exposed to yeast organisms every time you have sex. This exposure affects him in one of four different ways. First, even though your partner's mouth and/or genitalia are exposed to yeast, his body may simply rid itself of the yeast organisms.

Second, he may become a symptom-free carrier of yeast organisms. The initial exposure allows a yeast colony to establish itself on his body, but does so in a way that is totally harmless (and symptomless) to him. Yeasts may live in the foreskin crevasses (if he is not circumcised), in the opening at the tip of the penis, in the urethra, or in the penile fluids. In this case, even though he has no pain, itching, or inflammation, he may be serving as a yeast reservoir and routinely passing yeasts back to you. So his lack of symptoms should not be taken to mean that he is yeast-free. Penile colonization is four times more prevalent among male sexual partners of infected women than among men whose partners are not infected.

The third type of reaction your partner may experience to the exposure of yeasts is in the development of a mild rash. The penis becomes red and/or itchy shortly after intercourse. If the condition is mild and clears up easily and quickly, it is most likely an allergic reaction to the Candida organisms (if you are undergoing treatment, it could also be an allergic reaction to your preparation). An allergic reaction on the partner's part may indicate that he is being exposed to a significant number of yeast organisms and is a sign that cotreatment is appropriate. A rash that is hard to clear up or comes back frequently should be examined by a physician to make sure Candida is the correct diagnosis.

Finally, the most clear-cut indicator that yeast is a problem with your partner is if he actually develops a genital yeast infection. These are usually referred to as Candida balanitis or Candida balanoposthitis. Symptoms include penile reddening; dryness; itching; inflamed, weeping mucosal surfaces around the tip; and bright red spots, sometimes covered with white membranes. Candidal balanitis and balanoposthitis are sexually transmitted in most cases. About 80 percent of the female partners of infected men have positive yeast cultures. If your partner does have a yeast infection, it is extremely likely that you are also harboring significant numbers of yeast organisms yourself.

Providing specific information on partner cotreatment is difficult because so little research has been done in that area. About the only thing that is clear is that balanitis is more common in men living in tropical climates and in men who have not been circumcised. Given this, most clinicians recommend first that men pay extra attention to make sure the penis, foreskin, and genital area are always clean and dry. Uncircumcised men are more likely to transmit yeast infections simply because an uncircumcised penis is harder to clean well and yeasts can live comfortably under the foreskin. If your partner is uncircumcised, suggest that, when washing, he retract the foreskin and clean thoroughly. Even if he is circumcised, encourage him to clean and dry his genitalia and anus thoroughly at least twice a day. Changing underwear/trunks after swimming or sweating, and avoiding tight-fitting (especially synthetic) clothing for long periods, help keep the genitalia dry and cool.

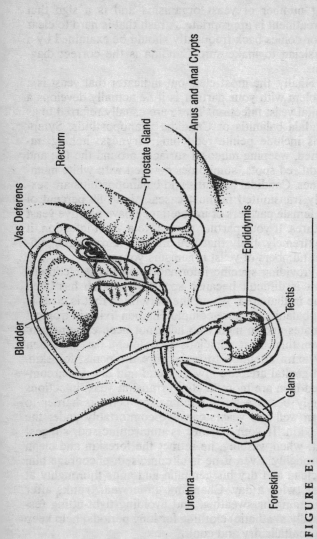

FIGURE E:
Cross-sectional view of male pelvic area

Bladder

Vas Deferens

Rectum

Prostate Gland

Anus and Anal Crypts

Epididymis

Testis

Glans

Foreskin

Urethra

Applying a topical antifungal cream to the penis and around the anus is the next line of attack. Any of the prescription antifungals work fine. Boric acid ointment also can be used for a nondrug antifungal. Have him wash his penile region and anus well. After drying, he should apply the cream to his whole penis and around the anus. Do this twice a day for four to five days. For maximum effectiveness, use an antifungal cream or suppositories on yourself once a day at the same time (making sure to use the cream around your anus as well). There is no evidence one way or the other about the effect of intercourse during treatment. Some practitioners suggest using a condom or abstaining from intercourse during the treatment period to avoid reinfection; other practitioners have even suggested ejaculation, away from your body, four to five times to clear out the prostate gland. Still a third group feels that, as long as intercourse is not physically uncomfortable, there is no benefit in curtailing sexual activity.

The final step in treating your partner is use of oral antifungals. The goal of the oral treatment is to lower the yeast population throughout your partner's body since women can be reinfected by a sexual partner who harbors Candida in the oral cavity or in the seminal vesicles which can pass on the fungus in semen at ejaculation. Oral antiyeast medication may prevent this. A three-week course of either nystatin or caprylic acid can be used for this purpose. More information on treatment of candidiasis can be found at the beginning of this chapter.

If the infection refuses to go away, it may be worth it for both of you to have a thorough genital examination and lab work in order to eliminate the possibility of an incorrect diagnosis or of multiple infections. If you have more than one partner, you should be regularly screened for sexually transmitted diseases (particularly nonspecific genital infection) as many of these diseases can coexist with Candida and have far more serious ramifications if left untreated.

If your partner is a woman, the odds of sexual transmissibility are low. If one partner is infected, however, there is a possibility that simple exposure to large numbers of yeast organisms may infect you. Again, cleanliness is the first line of attack. Local treatments (see Home Remedies and Antifungal Agents earlier in this chapter) are the second step. If both of you are experiencing constant reinfections, or if one of you is and there seems to be a relationship between sexual activity and yeast infections, then oral as well as local treatment for both of you is appropriate.

TREATMENT FOR SPECIAL CASES

Pregnancy

Candidal infections during pregnancy are the most troublesome of all vaginal yeast infections. Pregnancy is a time of extremely high susceptibility to yeast infections and is also the single most frequently cited opportunistic factor predisposing women to such infections. Not surprisingly, candidal vaginitis is the most frequent of all infections doctors report in maternity practice and occurs in pregnant women 10 to 20 times more frequently than in nonpregnant women. Once the infection appears, it is harder to eradicate, illustrating the fact that cure rates during pregnancy are much lower while recurrences are higher. Multiple courses of therapy are often required to achieve symptomatic relief.

Pregnancy-related yeast infections are nothing new; our grandmothers and their grandmothers were well aware that pregnancy was a time when a white, cheesy, itchy discharge occurred. That pregnancy indeed predisposes women to yeast susceptibility has been a proven fact for over 50 years. In 1937 the results of a study were released in which the vaginas of healthy women, pregnant and not, were inoculated with active yeast cultures and the group observed for subsequent yeast colonization and infection. Infection was induced in more than 80 percent of the pregnant women, but in only a minority of the nonpregnant women.

Pregnancy predisposes a woman to yeast infections primarily through hormonal changes, which in turn affect the overall body chemistry and alter the local vaginal environment. The higher levels of estrogen and progesterone associated with pregnancy produce an ample supply of sugars that promote yeast growth. As the hormones increase throughout the pregnancy, the incidence of yeast infection also increases to the time of delivery. The third trimester of pregnancy is the time when women are most at risk for impending infection.

In addition to the higher hormone levels, the pregnant woman faces higher caloric needs, particularly for protein and micronutrients like iron, calcium, and folic acid. Nature's way of protecting the developing fetus from malnutrition is by supplying it with nutritional reserves from mom. But if mom's diet is inadequate, the baby's needs will take priority. Mom may have mild nutritional deficiencies, making her much more susceptible to yeast infection. While pregnancy is the most cited factor in vaginal candidiasis, the second is pregnancy in malnourished mothers.

Making matters worse, it is when you are most susceptible to yeast infections that you have the fewest options for treatment. More importantly, during pregnancy, you are not only more susceptible to yeast infections, you are also more susceptible to being treated inappropriately or inadequately by the medical profession.

The fact that you have abundant white discharge

containing yeast colonies does not mean you require treatment. Additional discharge during pregnancy is normal. You only require treatment if you are uncomfortable with irritation, pain, or itching. Many doctors, all too eager to reach for their prescription pads, will begin treating you with antifungals upon visual observation of an increased discharge. Not only is this a waste of money and time, it may result in a misdiagnosis.

The time to be concerned about heavier discharge when you have no other symptoms is when there is a sudden profuse increase near the end of your pregnancy. Call your obstetrician/midwife anytime you have a noticeable change in discharge—in consistency or volume—near the end of a pregnancy. Also, after the twentieth week of the pregnancy, candidal vaginitis may be a sign to check your blood sugar levels; this requires a simple test that can be performed during your next doctor's visit.

If you are prone to yeast infection, you should be especially rigorous in taking preventative measures during pregnancy. Cut down on sugars, take multivitamins and multimineral tablets, supplement your gastrointestinal tract regularly with acidophilus, and keep the external genitalia and anal region clean and dry. The drier the vaginal area, the less hospitable it will be to yeast. Give it a few minutes to air out after a shower and carry a couple of changes of underwear with you or use panty liners and replace each one as it gets damp. (Refer to chapter 6 for more tips on prevention.)

If you do find yourself with a yeast infection, there are a number of treatment options although there is considerable disagreement on just what a pregnant woman should or shouldn't do. Physicians and midwives disagree among themselves as much as they do with each other. Check with your obstetrician/midwife before treating yourself and stick to the proven safe treatments. Typical nondrug options include acidophilus, yogurt, garlic, and homeopathic suppositories (used alone or in combination). Increase your garlic consumption in food and/or take garlic capsules. Pick up some acidophilus and take it daily. Garlic and acidophilus capsules as well as homeopathic suppositories can also be used directly in the vagina. Very gentle douching with yogurt using a thick mixture of half water, half yogurt may also help. (Stay far away from both povidone-iodine and gentian violet during pregnancy.) Your symptoms can be controlled adequately for a number of months with home remedies and, if needed, local antifungals. There is no need to rush into oral antifungal therapy provided you have the right diagnosis as vaginal candidiasis is usually self-limiting in pregnancy.

Of the prescription treatment options, local application of either nystatin and miconazole (in creams and suppositories) are your best bet. These can both be used when breast-feeding as well. Bear in mind that the first trimester (up to week 14) is the most crucial part of a pregnancy, that drugs taken at this time can have effects we don't know about or understand. Though nystatin and miconazole are considered safe for use in pregnancy, use them intelligently and attentively, and only after all other options are exhausted during the first trimester. Of these two prescription drugs, miconazole appears to be more effective than nystatin. Though both drugs have lower cure rates in pregnant women, nystatin's efficacy drops to near 50 percent. Two or three courses of therapy may be required if your infections fail to respond to the initial course.

Oral nystatin probably won't do you any harm if you're pregnant, but like all drugs, it is best avoided, if possible. Ketoconazole, creams and pills, should never be taken during pregnancy or while breast-feeding.

The bad news is that, for women predisposed to yeast infections, pregnancy may be a time when the infections flare up with the condition becoming more deeply entrenched after the baby arrives. Some women who have had little or no trouble with yeast infections will find that they now have frequent infections, the pregnancy serving as the vehicle for the condition to become established.

The good news is that the majority of women who experience yeast infections during pregnancy will find that the condition simply goes away once the baby is born. The months of pregnancy may have been a problematic period of chronic infections, but the situation will correct itself in the postpartum weeks with no intervention whatsoever.

Yeast and Infants

Newborns are the most helpless creatures in the world at birth. Not only do they require extensive caretaking, but they require it for much longer than the young of any other species. One important facet of their vulnerable state is that infants are not born with a fully developed immune system. It takes 18 months to two years of healthy growth for their immune system to mature.

In their early months, all infants, but especially those malnourished or with low birth weights, are extremely susceptible to pathogens in their environment, of which abundant yeast is a prime example. Not surprisingly, fungal infections in infants are not uncommon. Even in the absence of any predisposing factors, yeasts are able to seize upon a tempting opportunity: babies with sweet, warm, dark, moist crevices and limited disease-fighting defenses.

Yeast infections in infants manifest themselves in

two primary conditions: diaper rash and oral thrush. Each is discussed below.

Diaper Rash

Diaper rash is a term commonly used to describe eruptions occurring on the skin normally covered by a diaper. The trigger for diaper rash may be nothing more than constant warm wetness on tender skin. A baby's skin is extra sensitive, especially in the early months; loose or irritating bowel movements will exacerbate soreness around the anus and increase the likelihood of diaper rash.

Diaper rash is a common affliction, which generally looks like small areas of small bright red spots with patches of rough, red skin. If the rash is bad, raw spots and inflammation may develop.

While there are a handful of culprits responsible for diaper rash, Candida albicans is a common cause. Candida yeasts get to the baby's buttocks after passing through the child's gastrointestinal tract and exiting the body via the anus. Candida albicans cannot survive on human skin without the presence of moisture and warmth; this, however, does not pose a problem since most infants' anal regions are kept under the tight wrap of a moisture- and stool-retaining diaper 24 hours a day.

A slight diaper rash may develop and clear up readily by itself and this should be no cause for concern. If a rash is persistent or becomes inflamed, though, don't ignore it. Diaper rash can make the baby uncomfortable when sitting, moving, or getting a diaper changed. Urinating can be particularly painful.

The best preventative measure to avoid diaper rash is to keep the skin dry, for yeast cannot survive without moisture. A common practice the world over is simply to let the baby air out. If it is not warm enough to expose your baby to the sun without clothes, you can leave the diaper off for a few hours and let the skin breathe. Place old towels or cloth diapers (or use disposable bed pads available from your drugstore) in a warm room and let your child enjoy being naked for a while.

Another useful practice for keeping the little one dry is frequent diaper changing. Changing the diaper soon after it becomes wet will help prevent diaper rash from ever getting started. Applying baby powder to the diaper area regularly also helps absorb moisture and is a safe and inexpensive way to foster dryness. Use talc, not cornstarch. Like all starches, cornstarch breaks down into sugars that provide a good culture media for the yeasts. Caldesene medicated powder (4 oz. sells for $4.29) combines talc with calcium undecylenate to kill fungus and bacteria while keeping the skin dry. It can be used to clear up a rash or even as part of your baby's daily dressing and changing routine. Discontinuing the use of waterproof pants for the duration of the rash will also help promote dryness.

Once moisture is under control, the next step is to minimize the baby's exposure to yeasts. Yeast contamination of the diapers is not usually a problem if you are using disposables or cloth diapers from a diaper service (they sterilize their diapers with each washing). If you are using cloth diapers and washing at home, try using the hot cycle and/or drying the diapers on the highest heat setting to destroy unwanted microorganisms. Residue from laundry detergents can also lead to diaper rash so use only unscented, unperfumed soaps, like Ivory, Dreft, or Unscented Tide. Double rinsing can also help remove any detergent residue. A cup of bleach added to the water before putting in the clothing is a readily available and inexpensive antiseptic. By the same token, warm sunshine is a potent destroyer of many microorganisms. If the weather is nice, hang the diapers, bedclothes, and blankets out in the sun. Take the baby out for air, too.

Take care not to irritate the baby's skin. Never use alcohol or any harsh chemicals on reddened or inflamed skin. You may want to apply a gentle, nonperfumed cream (such as Calendula cream) to help relieve the irritation. When washing the baby, use a mild soap, warm water, and a soft washcloth. Be sure to rinse off all the soap, as leftover dried soap can also cause irritation.

Diaper rashes occur for all sorts of reasons and all are not necessarily caused by your diapering routine. Malnourished children get them more frequently than well-nourished children. Also, diaper rash sometimes means that your baby has food allergies, perhaps to a particular formula or to cow's milk products. Try changing formulas and, if still breast-feeding, cutting milk products from both your diets. You can replace them with soy formulas and/or goat's milk products. This will help you ascertain if the rash is an indicator of an allergic reaction. If the child is eating solid food, try reducing sugar intake; babies do not need sweets. Dilute juices by half with water and substitute low sugar snacks from your health food store (like crackers, rice cakes, and cookies sweetened only with fruit juice for cookies and sweets). Check the ingredients on the label of the brand of baby food you're using; many of these products contain large quantities of sugar. As long as you're looking, avoid the products with high salt content as well. Cutting back on sugar consumption will not only help in the treatment of diaper rash, but might also moderate mood swings, shifts in energy levels, and set a good precedent for a lifetime of healthy eating.

Some of the same home remedies for your yeast infection also work against diaper rash. Try applying an acidophilus paste (made by mixing the contents of a few capsules or some powder with a little water into a paste) to the infected areas. You can also coat the area with a gentle nonperfumed cream; try Calendula cream, made from the calendula flower (discussed earlier in this chapter). Gently rub the cream onto the inflamed areas several times a day.

If your baby's diaper rash persists after those remedies, there are a number of prepared products available. In the baby section of the drugstore you will find several creams for relief from diaper rash. Desitin and A&D are two common ones, costing about $3.50 for 2 ounces. These are vitamin-rich soothing creams that are generally effective even though they contain no antifungal agents. If the condition requires something stronger, use Gyne-Lotrimin or Monistat, the over-the-counter vaginal creams (each costing about $22.00 for a 45 gram tube) or check out the athletic section of the drugstores. Desenex, Tinactin, Micatin, and Lotrimin AF are athlete's foot creams (they cost about $7.00 for a 0.5 ounce tube), and are also antifungal creams. Mycolog II cream (made by Squibb) is the most commonly used prescription medication. Mycolog II contains a combination of nystatin to counteract the fungal infection and a cortisone to help remove the pain and tenderness. Available in 15, 30, 60, and 120 gram tubes, Mycolog II costs from $14.90 for the smallest tube to $75.00 for the large size. Check with your pharmacist to see if they carry any of these medications in a generic brand, which is usually less expensive. Creams should be rubbed in gently, but thoroughly, twice daily, applied to the entire inflamed area and all around the anus. Use as long as the inflammation persists and for a week after.

These preparations should only be used to treat the infection, not daily for weeks on end or as part of routine baby care. Keep these medications away from both your and the baby's eyes. Call the doctor if the infection has not cleared up within four days. If the rash does not begin to clear within a few days, or if the baby develops a fever with the rash, call the doctor right away. It may be something other than a yeast inflammation, and prompt medical attention is prudent.

Finally, time is always the best cure. As the baby gets older, the incidence and severity of diaper rash lessens.

Oral Thrush

Oral thrush is a mild fungal infection of the mouth. The patches of milky scum that coat the cheeks, tongue, and roof of the mouth make it look like the baby's mouth is covered with a permanent layer of yogurt. Even though it seems as if you could just wipe them away, the milky patches are firmly attached. The underlying skin may be inflamed and will occasionally bleed. (When you check your baby for oral thrush, be aware that the inner sides of the gums, where the upper molar teeth will eventually grow, are normally very pale. You can mistake it for thrush, but it is nothing to worry about.)

Vaginal yeast infections predominantly occur in women of childbearing years, while oral thrush crops up most often in infants and older folks, especially denture-wearers. While the incidence of vaginal yeast infection is increasing steadily, infant oral thrush on the whole has dropped dramatically. An 1838 textbook on pediatric medicine devoted fully one-third of its pages to thrush, and outbreaks in hospital wards and orphanages were common. Today, oral thrush does not even justify its own chapter in many pediatric texts and, while still common, it is easily controlled and therefore less likely to spread wildly.

As with diaper rash, the main factor in susceptibility to oral thrush in infants is their immature immune system. That less effective immune system combined with the mouth's dark, warm, moist, sweet environment, and you can understand why yeasts find the oral cavity a hospitable home. In older persons, a weakened immune system is also a factor; and in denture-wearers, it is the tiny nicks and abrasions to the oral membranes caused by the denture plates that are a common trigger.

Oral thrush may look fairly harmless, but it should not be ignored. It can be quite painful for the child. That pain, in turn, can mean the baby eats insufficient meals, cries and fusses, and can become dehydrated, and lose sleep.

Preventative care includes sterilizing the bottles and nipples as well as any pacifiers. Wash them in hot water and soap or run them through the dishwasher, which does a fine job of sterilizing. Besides reducing the baby's exposure from the feeding bottle, you will want to make sure your own nipples are not a source of infection since the sugars in breast milk and the warm, moist environment both facilitate yeast growth. Applying an antifungal ointment to the breast is an easy method of clearing this up; try Tinactin, Desenex, Gyne-Lotrimin, or Monistat, or, by prescription, try Monistat Derm, 15 grams for $14.90. Another easy over-the-counter technique is to apply Orithrush Mouthwash, from Ecological Formulas (available in health food stores). 8 ounces sell for $12.95.

Once you've reduced the baby's exposures to yeast, another trick is to give the baby half an ounce of fully cooled boiled water after a feeding. This washes the milk out of the mouth, which in turn reduces the nutrients there on which the fungus live.

If the child requires treatment, the most common approach (worldwide) is painting the yeast patches with gentian violet. The baby's mouth will get tinged blue, but this fades quickly. A 30 cc bottle of gentian violet sells for $2.95. Use a half teaspoon of gentian violet to four ounces of warm water. Apply the solution to each side of the cheek four times a day using an old dropper.

If your primary care provider recommends a prescription medication, your options include Nystex Oral Suspension from Savage ($12.45 for 60 ml) and Mycostatin Oral Suspension from Squibb ($28.50 for 60 ml). Ask your pharmacist if there is a generic nystatin oral suspension available at a lower cost. The oral suspensions are essentially the same: pleasant tasting, ready-to-use liquid formulations containing nystatin. They are specifically designed for the treatment of oral thrush and are safe for infants. Infants should receive two ml (200,000 units) four times a day; make sure you put one ml in each side of the mouth. The preparations all include a calibrated dropper for easy administration. The goal is to have the child hold the liquid in the mouth as long as possible before swallowing. One oddity to note is that these preparations contain sugar to make them palatable to the child. Fully 50 percent of the oral suspension is sugar. The destructive effect of the nystatin on the pathological yeast is designed to more than compensate for the growth-promoting effect of the sugar, but considering the cost and the sugar, gentian violet should be your first course of action.

Oral thrush responds quickly and easily to treatment and should be cleared up completely within four days. It's a good idea, though, to continue using the medications for at least 48 hours after the infection has subsided. Reported side effects are uncommon, but may include nausea, vomiting, bloating, gas, and diarrhea. If your baby does have a reaction, cut the dosage in half.

The occurrence of oral thrush, like diaper rash,

diminishes as the child gets older, especially as most infants who get it are still being fed primarily milk or formula. If the child has begun to eat, be sure to keep an eye on the sugar intake, high levels of which are a sure invitation to yeast.

TREATMENTS OF THE FUTURE

As always, science marches on, searching for better answers to our problems. Yeast researchers around the globe are actively researching new remedies for diseases associated with fungal colonization. The AIDS crisis has served to accelerate that research since AIDS-infected patients, with their weakened immune systems, are particularly susceptible to yeast colonization.

It would be wonderful to report that scientists are well on their way to developing a magic pill or vaccine for candida vulvovaginitis. Who wouldn't welcome the announcement of a safe, quick, effortless "magic bullet" to eradicate yeast infections once and for all. Since chronic yeast infection has more to do with the host's body being compromised than with a specific pathogen, this is unlikely.

What does the future hold? Certainly, we can look forward to some new antifungal drugs for both oral and topical use. Most likely, new delivery vehicles will also be introduced, allowing for shorter and shorter treatment times and convenient timed-release dosages.

Inexpensive home test kits for diagnosing a variety of conditions are increasingly available to consumers, though it is unlikely that a reliable home test for Candida will emerge as the kit would have to ascertain whether the Candida organisms were causing an infection or just residing peacefully in the vagina. However, it is likely that home test kits will become available that could rule out other causes of vaginitis, making home treatment of suspected candidiasis less risky. New methods for analyzing both vaginal odors and secretions could translate into home test kits for bacterial vaginitis, chlamydia, trichomoniasis, and gonorrhea. Tests utilizing dipsticks, to test pH levels, and potassium hydroxide, to detect characteristic odors in vaginal secretions, could be made available at low cost. The elimination of specific diseases would allow women to know right away if there was a risk to delaying medical treatment.

One benefit of the boom in home testing is the increased information that goes hand-in-hand with the marketing of these kits to consumers. Informative directions and fact sheets, as well as nurse-staffed, toll-free telephone numbers, all help educate the public on what to look for and what danger signs to monitor.

Two other likely approaches are hormonal manipulation and bacterial manipulation. One future treatment using hormonal manipulation involves injecting a long-acting progesterone (Depo-Provera is currently being tested in Australia) into the body; this appears to substantially reduce a woman's susceptibility to recurrent vulvovaginal candidiasis. The effectiveness of the treatment would be limited, however, to nonpregnant women of childbearing age because pregnancy and estrogen supplementation (used by menopausal and postmenopausal women) appear to counteract the positive effects of the drug. Various other kinds of hormonal manipulation will likely be explored through the 1990s (including the use of injectable hormones for contraceptive protection), and there is every reason to expect promising results.

Another focus of Candida research is manipulation of bacteria to build up the body's natural resistance to yeast infection. One researcher has used lactobacilli vaccines in the treatment of female genital infections. A cure, or at least the marked improvement of symptoms, occurred in 80 percent of the women. Less invasive than a vaccine, another potential treatment approach is yeast infection prophylactics. Suppositories or creams containing healthy bacteria, lactobacilli, and/or other yeast fighters, could be used before an infection appears. Use of such a product concurrent with antibiotic use or in conjunction with the menstrual cycle could prevent an infection from ever getting established. Bacterial therapy poses a potential for short treatment times, limited mess, and no side effects.

As the scientific world continues to unravel the mysteries of fungi, the good news is that our ability to control these miraculous organisms will undoubtedly continue to grow. The bad news is that the incidence of yeast infections has grown steadily in the latter half of this century due to many of the previous "advances" of our society. As we continue to advance in our medical knowledge, so, too, may we better understand the nature of the yeast organism and develop ways to coexist harmoniously.

6

֍

STAYING FREE

•

> Vaginitis is your body speaking to you. It's important to listen to your body and look at what's happening in the rest of your life.
>
> —*Medical Self-Care*, summer 1983

*P*revention is still the best way to avoid illness. Yeast organisms live harmlessly all around us, present in almost all living organisms; they only cause illness when the body's ability to fight disease becomes compromised. Given this simple fact, yeast infections can be greatly reduced simply by safeguarding your good health. Your time and energy are much better spent maintaining your health than curing yourself once you've become sick.

By taking an active role in changing your diet, clothing, hygiene, and leisure time, you can prevent the infections before they ever get started. If an infection takes you by surprise, however, you can use prescriptions and home remedies to ease the irritation and reduce the discharge and inflammation, giving you a physical and mental breather as you begin tackling the yeast situation. While most prescriptions and home remedies are fine for relief from symptoms, the only way to end the cycle of infection permanently is by maintaining your healthy status.

The fact that your body has become infected with yeast is a sign that something is wrong, your internal disease-fighting ability has been reduced or altered. Because the ultimate treatment is to rebuild and regain full health and vitality, you should not view prevention as something to be practiced for a few days each month, before your period, or only when you take antibiotics; rather, prevention should be a part and parcel of your daily life.

Some women are prone to allergies, others to headaches, and others to yeast infections. As we have seen, genetic factors, poor nutrition, multiple pregnancies, frequent doses of antibiotics, or some other combination of events may all play a part in this susceptibility. All types of women may be affected. Indeed, vaginal yeast infections can strike women of all ages, races, economic classes (wealthy women can be hard hit because they go to doctors the most frequently where prescriptions for antibiotics are common), geographic locations (hot, humid climates are the worst), and levels of sexual activity (from virgins to prostitutes).

To start to remedy your own situation examine what factors in your life most likely led you down this particular path (chapter 2 discusses the major factors). Then you will be ready to take the necessary steps to remove or reduce them. Stress may trigger an infection in some; in others it may be too much sugar. Some women get them with every menstrual cycle. Modify those situations that you can (e.g., substitute narrow-spectrum antibiotics for broad-spectrum, go off the Pill, cut down on sweets). Once yeast is entrenched in your body, removing the trigger is just the first of many steps. Still, what you do in an overall effort to help your body in its task of keeping you vibrant and healthy can be critical.

If your infections are irregular and easily controlled, you may never need the tips in chapter 5. The information in this chapter, however, can help you remain infection-free. Your goal should be to provide your body with all the tools it needs to perform well 365 days a year. The advice below is to help you increase your general state of wellness, leaving you less susceptible to infections of all sorts.

General Prevention Tips

In America today, well over $200 billion is spent each year on doctors, hospitals, and medical care. Hundreds of millions of prescriptions are written annually. Though medical care can help alleviate illness, control disease, or provide treatment, it does not guarantee long-term health. To a great extent, what keeps us healthy or unhealthy is the way in which we live our daily lives—what we eat; how often we exercise; how much rest we get; what kind of stresses we face; whether we consume alcohol, cigarettes, or drugs; what kinds of jobs we have; whether we find satisfaction and joy in our relationships. By taking greater responsibility for our health, we can reduce both the severity and the frequency of illness.

Lifestyle decisions are very important; according to recent government studies, fully 80 percent of all cancer may be related to the environment and to things we eat, drink, and smoke, rather than to factors we cannot control such as our genetic makeup. More and more, people are avoiding caffeine and alcohol. Smoke-free environments are fast becoming the standard, rather than the exception. Excellent athletic clothing and facilities are widely available throughout the country. Supermarkets and health food stores stock a large selection of fresh and wholesome foods year-round. Fast-food establishments offer baked potatoes and salad bars as alternatives to fat-laden, highly processed meals.

Every body is unique. Scientists are finding that although we humans share many similarities, each body has its own biochemical individuality. There are certain things we all require to survive, a minimum level of nutrients and enough exercise so that our muscles do not atrophy. Our bodies' needs also differ. Some people enjoy shellfish; it makes others break out in hives. Some people seem to thrive on chocolate; others experience a reaction to it. The same holds true for milk, wheat, nuts, berries, etc. Some people just start to feel alive after running six miles, others find running to be tedious and injurious at best. A good mechanic learns through trial and error the needs of each individual car, and eventually these needs become intuitive. The more you become sensitive and responsive to your body's specific needs, the closer you will be to achieving not only consistent and reliable, but peak performance.

FUEL FOR YOUR BODY

Most of the plants around us have green leaves. Green plants make their own food; producing it from the air, soil, water, and sunlight. But the *sole source* of energy production for our bodies comes from food intake; it only makes sense to provide ourselves with the best possible foods to fuel our systems. It is essential that we receive certain building blocks to sustain life. In past centuries sailors severely deprived of vitamin C died of scurvy; goiter, beriberi, and pellagra resulted from extreme deficiencies of iodine, thiamine, and vitamin B3, respectively. Today we know that mineral deficiencies of calcium, potassium, and selenium contribute to osteoporosis, cancer, and heart disease. These diseases occur in the extreme, but minor deficiencies also affect human performance.

The best single way of getting the proper nutrients is by eating a balanced diet. Fresh, wholesome foods are broken down by our bodies into the building blocks we need to maintain a nutritional balance. Highly refined, processed foodstuffs, while providing calories, do not provide the necessary building blocks, which have been removed or destroyed in the processing, and often are short of micronutrients. Pay attention to the nutritional value of the foods you eat. Just changing a few of your cooking and eating habits can make a big difference between consuming nutrients and consuming empty calories. For example, steaming vegetables rather than frying or boiling them preserves many of the natural nutrients. Substitute a piece of fruit for chips with your next sandwich; snack on cheese and crackers instead of a candy bar in the afternoon; drink soda water with lime or fruit juice instead of soda pop for a cool refreshing drink; order your sandwich on whole wheat bread instead of white.

The vast majority of Americans can afford to eat almost any diet, yet choose to consume about 60 percent of daily caloric intake in highly refined, preserved, and fortified foods. This diet is so deficient in dietary fiber that physicians end up writing millions of prescriptions annually for laxative preparations. The following suggestions are good general guidelines to nourish your body and reduce the likelihood of yeast infections.

• Significantly reduce your intake of sugars, especially refined sugar. Yeasts thrive when their hosts consume a diet high in sugars, such as foods containing sugar, corn syrup, honey, molasses, and other sweeteners. These sugars not only alter normal metabolism, they also radically change the normal pH of the vagina.

When yeasts are fed sugar, they convert it into carbon dioxide, resulting in fermentation; without sugar, yeast production is severely curtailed. Many women find that a candy binge will often result in a yeast infection, others need only overdo their fruit intake to find that the yeast enjoyed the snack as much as they did.

It is ironic that the messages your body sends you are not necessarily in your best interest. Responding to sugar cravings premenstrually, during pregnancy, when taking antibiotics, or when under extra stress is exactly the wrong thing to do. These are times when your body is already vulnerable to an infection—the last thing you want to do is make it more likely to happen. To minimize the effects of sugar, consume it as part of a meal.

Dietary Guidelines for Americans Issued by the U.S. Department of Agriculture and the U.S. Department of Health and Human Services, 1985.

To Avoid Too Much Sugar

- Use less of all sugars and foods containing large amounts of sugars, including white sugar, brown sugar, raw sugar, honey, and syrups. Examples include soft drinks, candies, cakes, and cookies.
- Remember, how often you eat sugar and sugar-containing food is as important to the health of your teeth as how much sugar you eat. It will help to avoid eating sweets between meals.
- Read food labels for clues on sugar content. If the name sugar, sucrose, glucose, maltose, dextrose, lactose, fructose, or syrups appears first, then there is a large amount of sugar.
- Select fresh fruits or fruits processed without syrup or with light, rather than heavy syrup.

Become aware of the sugar content of what you eat, read labels and remember that foods like molasses and dried fruits have high sugar content even though the label does not list "sugar." Similarly, cornstarch, sucrose, and fructose are all sugars. Try snacking on carrot sticks, chewing gum, or sucking on something sour when the sugar cravings hit. One encouraging note is that many women who have had severe sugar cravings (especially premenstrually) report that as they respond less to the cravings, their bodies demand less sugar, so that the struggle to avoid sugar is one that may be intense, but short-lived.

• Make a point of eating fresh vegetables, fruits, meat, and fish, in their natural states, not canned, preserved, processed, precooked, sugared, or salted. In many processed foods, the required heating and addition of chemicals destroys the nutritional base. In general, the longer the shelf life of a product, the more it has been processed and refined, the less likely it is to contribute to your health. If many of the foods you consume (excluding grains and nuts) do not spoil when left overnight on the kitchen counter, you may not be eating enough raw, unprocessed foods. If you can't eat fresh foods all the time, dried or frozen are the next best from a nutritional point of view.

• Eat raw foods each day. Many people eat so many meals out of deep fat fryers, aluminum cans, or microwave ovens, they don't even realize they're not eating anything raw. Eat fresh, green salads, fruits, vegetables, nuts, and seeds; they are loaded with nutrients and also provide you with natural fiber in its original form.

• Eat a variety of foods and rotate them regularly. It's easy to fall into food ruts: cereal for breakfast, sandwich and chips for lunch, pizza and beer for dinner. Try not to rely on the same foods all the time. The National Research Council recommends eating six or more servings of fruits and vegetables, as well as six servings of breads or cereals each day, just to get the right amounts and types of dietary fiber. Clearly, consuming a variety of foodstuffs is the easiest way to fill in any nutritional gaps in our diet. Seeking variety also makes you more aware of what you are consuming and gives you a good excuse to try things you might otherwise shy away from.

In addition, some people have found it valuable to rotate their foods as a way of minimizing the effects of subtle food allergies, which can develop when one kind of food is eaten very frequently. Subtle or hidden food allergies occur when you have a sensitivity to a certain foodstuff, but the reaction is not immediately apparent, as it might be with seafood, for instance. Low-level food allergies may be affecting your health at a low, but often chronic level. Common offenders include milk, cheese, wheat, corn, and soy, though any food can be a problem. Testing for such food sensitivities is difficult at best and usually involves the elimination of suspect foodstuffs from your diet for four days, then monitoring your body for an elevated pulse, some physical or emotional reaction, or skin sensitivity, as you reintroduce each isolated food. See Appendix C: Suggested Reading for references to explore this further.

• Eat three meals a day. Your body needs a regular source of energy (calories). Allowing time to digest those calories will help you realize their maximum value. Since the enzymes in saliva are essential to the process of breaking down foodstuffs, eating on the run, while standing, not chewing your food thoroughly, and skipping meals reduces the benefits of food. Eat in a relaxed environment as often as possible, as relaxation aids digestion.

• Try to restrict your fat intake. Although our bodies need fat, as a society we consume too much. The typical American consumes 35 to 38 percent of

Dietary Guidelines for Americans Issued by the U.S. Department of Agriculture and the U.S. Department of Health and Human Services.

To Avoid Too Much Fat, Saturated Fat, and Cholesterol

- Choose lean meat, fish, poultry, and dry beans and peas as protein sources.
- Use skim and low-fat milk and milk products.
- Moderate your use of egg yolks and organ meats.
- Limit your intake of fats and oils, especially those high in saturated fat, such as butter, cream, lard, heavily hydrogenated fats (some margarines), shortenings, and foods containing palm and coconut oils.
- Trim fat off meats.
- Broil, bake, or boil rather than fry.
- Moderate your use of foods that contain fat, such as breaded and deep-fried foods.
- Read labels carefully to determine both amount and type of fat present in foods.

---

daily caloric intake from fat. The U.S. Surgeon General's guidelines suggest reducing that percentage to 30. Cut down on butter and oil, buy cheese and meat with a lower fat content, and minimize the fried foods that you eat. Since heat alters the fat molecules, try to consume fats not prepared with a heat process, such as butter or cold pressed oils (the label will tell you if it is cold pressed).

• Tobacco, alcohol, and caffeine are all addictive substances that should be minimized or eliminated. Caffeine wreaks havoc on your body's blood sugar levels, sending them up and down (and your mood with it) within minutes of ingestion. Soon your body doesn't know what it wants. Addictive drugs do more harm than good, sending you signals based on the chemical addiction rather than on the real needs of your body. If you don't feel you can eliminate them, cut them back drastically and regulate your consumption so that you are in control, rather than the other way around.

• Be sure to get enough fiber. You want foods to pass through your body, not stay there and incubate. The United States is a constipated nation, in large part due to a diet severely lacking in fiber. The laxative business, both prescription and over-the-counter, rings up hefty profits as a result. Fiber is not only an important component of a good health regimen, it is also an important preventative measure for colon cancer. If you find that you need help staying regular, increase your fluid intake. Vegetables, fruits, and grain products are the main sources for dietary fiber. Additionally, try natural fiber such as psyllium husks (available in health food stores), bran, or prune juice, all of which relieve constipation.

• Drink plenty of fluids. The time-tested advice for most illnesses, from colds to bladder infections, is to drink fluids. It's good advice for healthy people, too. Most of us do not drink enough. It doesn't have to be plain water: herbal teas, soda water, natural juice drinks, vegetable juices, and soups all count. When fluids pass through your system, they help flush out present and potential problems. Every time you see a drinking fountain, stop and have a drink while counting to 10. You should not, however, drink heavily 15 minutes before, during, or shortly after meals. Drinking with meals may dilute the digestive juices and may prevent you from getting the full nutritional value out of your foods.

• Take a regular vitamin and mineral supplement if your food sources are not adequate or are highly refined. The preferred source of vitamins and minerals is your food. But no food is grown under optimal conditions. Even the fresh products have often spent long periods between the farm and your fork, whether in a truck or sitting in a supermarket. And many of the fresh foods available, such as meat and vegetables, have been treated with pesticides, preservatives, hormones, radiation, dyes, and antibiotics. Stress taxes your body. Try taking an extra vitamin a few days before your period and anytime you are under extra stress. Even with the most sincere effort, it is difficult to eat the proper proportions of carbohydrates, proteins, and fats every day.

Scientists are finding that vitamins play a greater role than previously thought in inhibiting disease. A good vitamin and mineral supplement may provide substances lacking in your diet. Supplements, as the name suggests, should be used to make up for lacks in your daily diet rather than be used as an alternative to eating well. Fortunately, good quality supplements are widely available, and have a high degree of safety. (Some people are sensitive to consumed yeasts, so choose a brand that says yeast-free.) Ask your primary care giver or health food store for a suggestion.

Is diet really that important? Absolutely. Enhanced susceptibility to Candida infections and higher death rates due to *C. albicans* have been shown in rats deficient in certain vitamins. The normal digestive tract maintains a small but constant yeast population. According to Dr. Sidney M. Baker, under normal conditions, diet markedly affects the total number of yeast organisms present; a person may start out being susceptible to an overgrowth of yeast because of a subtle imbalance brought about by suboptimal diet; once begun, the cycle is self-perpetuating.

EXERCISE

Lack of regular exercise ranks as the next largest factor causing poor health in our society. In the largest and most exhaustive study on the subject (over 13,000 men and women), the Institute for Aerobics Research recently found that even a moderate amount of exercise—taking a daily half-hour walk—significantly reduces the incidence of heart disease and other illnesses. In addition to the cardiovascular and muscular benefits of exercise, the participants also benefitted from an increase in bowel motility.

Many people who once thought of exercise as painful, tedious, and boring have come to enjoy it as a means of managing tension, spending time with family and friends, and feeling better. Everybody requires exercise to reach an optimum state of health and wellness.

A regular fitness program helps you to:

- maintain a strong heart and build up healthy lungs, muscles, and bones;
- enhance overall physical, mental, and emotional well-being as you reduce the tension and stresses of life;
- increase your energy level and the overall performance of your body;
- get the sleep you need to recharge yourself each day.

Exercise is truly a gift you give yourself. Fitness cannot be bought or borrowed, faked or stolen; no one can do it for you. Getting in shape is something you must do for yourself, a commitment you make to taking care of your body and your mind. And there is nothing better to improve your perspective on life—office politics, marital spats, even financial pressures never look quite so gruesome after a vigorous workout.

Everyone can find an activity that is right for them. Exercise can be done with no other equipment than a good pair of shoes, in the privacy of your own home, in a club with instructors and facilities, just about anywhere. YMCAs and YWCAs all over the country offer low-cost facilities and instruction. Whether it is walking, bicycling, judo, tennis, yoga, swimming, or aerobics, find something that interests you and stick with it. Make a commitment with yourself today to get into a regular habit of exercise and, if possible, combine it with fresh air, sunshine, and companionship.

Exercise doesn't have to interrupt your schedule. You can exercise with your kids: Sign them up on a neighborhood soccer team then sign yourself up as a referee. Try meeting a business colleague at the gym instead of the bar. Go for a bike ride with your date instead of sitting in a movie. Chat with your friends while walking in a park instead of over coffee. Buy a stationary bicycle or rowing machine and work out during the evening news. Getting in shape is a matter of attitude; when exercise is an integral part of life, rather than a burden and inconvenience, you'll find that it does fit in. And remember, beginning is the hardest. Once you've begun, the feeling is addictive, literally: when the body works hard, it produces a substance called endorphins, which actually make you feel good.

STRESS AND WARNING FLAGS

A great deal has been written about stress. We all have stress in our lives. Some people have demands pulling them in all directions at once and love it. Others have little tolerance for the demands of anyone or anything. The bottom line, though, is your own subjective judgment.

If you feel you have too much stress, it's time to

figure out what to do about it. It may be that your body just cannot cope physically. It may be that there is too much happening in your emotional, family, or work life, and you need to seek outside help to sort it out. Maybe you aren't getting any time to yourself and need to find that regular space that is yours, alone, to spend any way you wish.

Whatever the reason, the warning flags of stress should be taken seriously. Chronic fatigue, dramatic mood swings, premenstrual syndrome, addiction to a drug or substance, constant hyperventilation, a multitude of seemingly unrelated health problems, regular feelings of anger, fantasies of violence—all these are signs that your life is not in order.

Sit down and figure out some solutions because warning flags are just that: warnings. Attend to them now while the choice is still yours. It may help to follow the advice we all received when learning to cross the street: Stop, Look, and Listen.

Summary of General Prevention Tips

- reduce consumption of sugars
- increase consumption of fresh foods
- increase consumption of raw foods
- eat a balanced and varied diet
- chew your meals well
- reduce consumption of fats
- reduce or eliminate tobacco, alcohol, caffeine, and other addictive substances
- increase consumption of fiber
- increase consumption of fluids
- take a vitamin/mineral supplement daily, especially premenstrually
- get regular exercise
- try to minimize stress

Specific Prevention Tips

In addition to becoming aware of your nutritional and physical requirements, there are other specific things you can do to protect yourself against yeast infections.

GETTING OFF THE PILL

No woman who is susceptible to yeast problems should remain on the Pill. These contraceptive hormones are extraordinarily convenient; unfortunately, its effects are not limited to birth control.

The first suggestion that women who use oral contraceptives may be predisposed to vaginal candidiasis came in 1964. Further reports of "Pill-associated" vaginitis appeared soon after and have continued steadily, even with the lower dosage pills now available. Researchers have also reported that women taking the Pill respond less well to antifungal therapy, often requiring double or even triple antifungal prescriptions to clear an infection. In some cases, the Pill had to be discontinued before a cure could be achieved at all.

There are, however, thousands of women who seem to take the Pill for years with no side effects; still, women who suffer from recurrent bouts of vaginitis should explore alternative methods of birth control. Not only will your body benefit from getting off the Pill, but some other forms of birth control can actually help maintain the health of your vagina. The spermicides used with the diaphragm and sponge help acidify the environment while they dilute the vaginal yeast population. In addition, spermicides kill more than just sperm—they help protect you from a number of harmful organisms, such as yeast, gonorrhea, trichomonas, and maybe even the AIDS virus.

Each woman must decide what form of birth control is right for her. Many find that the diaphragm offers the most security, while others enjoy the convenience of the contraceptive sponge used with a condom. Your primary care giver should be happy to work with you in finding a suitable alternative that will both prevent pregnancy and discourage yeast growth.

VAGINAL CARE

The environment of the vagina is in delicate balance between dozens of different organisms. The normal, healthy vagina cleanses itself every day. Slight discharge from the cervix and vaginal walls keeps the vagina moist, and the downward flow of moisture carries old cells, menstrual blood, and other matter out quite effectively. In a normal, healthy woman, no intervention is required to maintain daily vaginal health.

Yeast infections can be triggered when there is enough of a disruption of the natural vaginal balance in favor of the yeasts. The vaginal environment is influenced by a number of factors, including hormonal levels, cleanliness, sexual activity, method of birth control, physical abrasions, chemical irritations, and stress.

VAGINAL pH

When the pH of the vagina goes above or below the normal range, potentially harmful organisms (for example, trichomonads) may flourish. Additionally, the lactobacilli organisms that live in the vagina and help control the yeast population prefer an acidic vaginal environment. Vaginal candidiasis is generally associated with a vaginal pH just slightly more alkaline than normal, although yeasts can thrive in a wide range of environments. Occasionally, it may be helpful to the body to readjust the vaginal pH back to its correct acidity to help it maintain its built-in defenses against opportunistic invaders.

Both sexual activity and menstruation can raise vaginal pH. Sexual arousal and orgasm alone, without intercourse, substantially increase vaginal pH. Seminal fluid is alkaline, typically 7.8, and can affect the vaginal environment for hours to days after intercourse. In addition, menstrual blood is also alkaline at around 7.0. During menstruation and at times of prolonged or frequent sexual activity, your body has to work hard to maintain its lower, normal vaginal pH. Paying extra attention to hygiene and ventilation at these times can reduce your susceptibility to problems of all sorts.

Douches should not be a regular activity, but an occasional douche when your susceptibility to infection is high, can be a good preventative measure to correct a pH imbalance before an infection occurs. Wearing a tampon, diaphragm, or sponge with a slightly acidic substance is another, perhaps more convenient, way to maintain acidity in the vagina. (See chapter 5 for information and instructions.)

IRRITATIONS/ABRASIONS

Normal healthy skin does not support a resident yeast population, but any damage to skin can lead to rapid colonization. Similarly, minor vaginal abrasions or local trauma allow yeast organisms a place to grow and flourish. Infrequent, but intense, sexual relations may precipitate a yeast infection. These can be seen regularly in women whose partners return after being away for an extended period (such as in military marriages), and in women beginning sexual relations with a new partner, especially after a long period of celibacy. The cause may be the introduction of yeast from the partner, but may also result from yeast growth in and around small abrasions occurring during vigorous sexual activity.

If your vagina is normally dry, if you've had a series of painful infections, or if you are resuming sexual activity after a break, you may want to use some extra lubrication. Even if your body normally produces plenty of lubrication, any tension during sex (including worrying about getting a yeast infection) will result in your body producing less lubrication than usual. Extra lubrication can make the difference between enjoyable sex and painful sex. You can use lubricated condoms or birth control creams and jellies; these products offer good lubrication and, to a limited extent, help destroy infectious organisms. Another good choice for lubrication is a water-soluble commercial sexual lubricant such as K-Y Jelly or Ortho Personal Lubricant (available in drugstores without prescription). Pure vegetable oil or coconut oil (available in health food stores) do not have the foul taste of spermicides and are inexpensive effective lubricants which can be used genitally as well as for body massage. Never use Vaseline or any petroleum jelly product as a lubricant; not only are these not sterile, but worse, they tend to remain in the vagina because they are difficult to wash away. In addition, any petroleum-based product will destroy the latex of condoms and diaphragms, reducing or eliminating the effectiveness of those for birth control.

Hygiene

Wash both your vulva and anus regularly using only pH balanced soaps (Dove has a lower pH than pure soap) or nonsoap cleansers (such as glycerine soaps). Pure soaps are not only alkaline, but are also very harsh on the skin. Pat yourself dry thoroughly using a dry, clean towel.

Wash and dry yourself well after swimming or athletic activities. The chlorine in pools can irritate the vagina and helps lead to yeast infections. Candida loves moisture; the organisms cannot survive at normal room humidity. Women who swim or work out in leotards or tight clothing should remove their damp clothing promptly after they finish exercising, wash or shower, then dry and change into loose cotton clothing.

It is important to keep anything that comes in contact with your vagina impeccably clean. If you use a diaphragm, menstrual sponge, vibrator, or dildo, douche equipment, wash them well after each use with warm water and a mild soap. Put them away in a protected place after they are thoroughly dry.

Always wipe your anus from front to back so that yeast from the anus won't get into the vagina or urethra. Never let anything (fingers, vibrators, penis, etc.) come into contact with your vagina once it has been in contact with your anus. The prevalence of Candida albicans in the rectal region is three to four times that of the vagina. It is generally assumed that, in some instances, the infestation spreads to the vagina from other sites, the anus being the most often implicated. Correct wiping and hygiene are especially important any time you have diarrhea or a loose stool.

Insufficiently sterilized diapers have been implicated as a source of reinfection in infants. Similarly, your own underwear may be one of your worst enemies. Four researchers in Britain decided to see if Candida albicans could survive on underwear after normal laundering and drying with standard household detergents. They designed a simulated laundering process using both cotton and nylon fabric. The results: Candida albicans was recovered from both types of fabric after this procedure using normal washing temperature (122°F). When the temperature was raised to 158°F, or if the clothes were ironed, the fungus could not be found. From this evidence, you may want to consider washing your underwear on the hot cycle or adding a bit of bleach to the load. Alternatively, drying your underclothes outside on a sunny day can also effectively eliminate any lingering yeast organisms.

Shower or bathe daily whenever possible. One study found that vaginitis occurred less frequently when a bath or shower was taken rather than with a "quick rinse down." One guess is that with a "rinse down," the yeasts are more easily transferred from the anus to the vagina, whereas in a more thorough, longer shower or bath they are washed away.

Never use feminine hygiene sprays. They offer no health benefits whatsoever and can be irritating or, worse, provoke an allergic reaction. Chemical irritations can also be caused by disinfectants in bathing water, vaginal deodorants, contraceptive foams and jellies, and even some soaps. Stop using any substance you suspect of causing a chemical irritation.

Make sure your sexual partner(s) are clean. Your partners should be as conscientious about personal hygiene as you. It is a good practice for a man to wash his penis daily since there is significant evidence that some women can be infected or reinfected with yeasts from a sexual partner. If you suspect a correlation between your infections and sexual activity, follow the guidelines in chapter 5 on treating the partner. If you or your male partner(s) are being treated for a genital infection, make sure he wears a condom during intercourse to minimize the transfer of an infection.

Tampons

A Danish study (1974) found a significant correlation between yeast infections and menstrual habits. The researchers found that women who rely on tampons during menstruation have candidiasis significantly less frequently than women using sanitary napkins only. Their explanation was that napkins become damp and stay damp, and that they close off the vaginal opening, creating a warm, moist, enclosed system for the yeast organisms to grow. They may also act as an infection link between the anus and the vagina. Another theory is that yeast organisms thrive in the higher pH of the vagina created by the menstrual blood and may actually feed off the blood.

Wear tampons during your period whenever possible. During heavy flows, two can be inserted (tie the strings together if you might forget you are wearing two—a forgotten tampon is a fertile source for infection of all sorts). During light flow, a diaphragm may be all that is needed to catch the blood. (This is also a handy way to make love without the mess during your period.) Putting a little spermicide on the diaphragm will help to lower the vaginal pH, since menstrual blood is more alkaline than the normal vaginal pH, and the spermicide will also provide additional lubrication. Just rinse it out a couple times a day and reinsert it. It can also be emptied while it is still inside by reaching a finger up just enough to break the seal to let the stored blood flow out. Clean your diaphragm regularly. Do not allow the blood to sit inside the diaphragm for more than six hours. Also, prescription antifungal preparations used when you are wearing a diaphragm may compromise the integrity of the latex rubber and should therefore be avoided when you're going to use your diaphragm.

The hormonal changes around the time of menstruation and the presence of menstrual blood with its many nutrients and high pH mean that you are particularly susceptible to yeast infections immediately before, during, and after menstruation. Precautions should be used most rigorously then. Using vinegar douches, for example, can help restore the proper pH.

You will want to wash and dry more often during menstruation, too, to remove the blood and ventilate the vagina.

CLOTHING

Yeast infections are a worldwide problem, particularly in tropical climates, with high heat and humidity and large consumption of sweet fruits. In the summer, heat and sweat provide yeast organisms with a great breeding ground. But, by wearing fabrics that do not breathe and thus close off the area, you might simulate this tropical environment around the vagina year-round. In the winter, layers of clothing can result in a nestlike breeding ground for yeast. Avoid any clothing that is tight in the thighs or crotch, especially those clothes made of nylon or synthetic fabrics and panty hose. While synthetic fabrics can be smooth, sleek, and sexy, they should never be worn snugly next to the skin.

One trick which has helped a great many women who wear panty hose regularly is to buy one of the brands with a separate cotton crotch insert (such as L'eggs Regular) and then to cut a hole the size of a quarter into the crotch piece. This allows the air to get in and moisture to get out without affecting the integrity of the stockings. Wearing stockings and a garter belt also solves this problem of closing.

Ideally, your vagina should always be clean and ventilated. Clean, dry cotton underpants should be worn. Be aware, though, that cotton holds onto moisture and wet cotton underwear is not going to help one bit. If you have a regular discharge, wear a thin panty shield and change it regularly. If you engage in sports or other sweaty activities, carry a change of underwear. The more you close up the body, the more you allow a self-supporting ecosystem to be maintained. Some women find that tap pants (stylish versions of men's jockey shorts) offer comfort and extra ventilation, and are therefore a nice alternative to skin-clinging underwear. Manufacturers of sports clothing are also beginning to offer underclothes made of breathable fabrics. These new fibers wisk moisture away from the skin so that it stays dry, much like disposable diapers. Gilda Marx makes a line of leotards and tights with such fabrics. Nighttime is an especially good opportunity to give your vagina a chance to breathe; sleep without any bottoms or wear loose cotton pajamas to give your vagina a chance to breathe.

Summary of Specific Prevention Tips

- stop using the Pill
- take antibiotics only if you must, then take only narrow-spectrum ones
- keep the vagina, vulva, and anus clean and dry
- douche occasionally with a mild vinegar solution, especially when sexually active and during menstruation
- use extra lubrication during sex
- wear loose, dry underclothing
- wash underwear in hot water, with an antiseptic, or sun dry
- do not use feminine hygiene sprays
- make sure your sexual partners are clean
- wear tampons instead of pads during menses but do not leave a tampon in for more than eight hours

The Yeast-Free Diet

The purpose of a yeast-free diet is twofold. One is diagnostic and the other is for treatment. The diagnostic use of a yeast-free diet helps people discover whether or not they are sensitive to yeasts. When used in this way, the diet should be followed quite strictly and . . . may often be ended by a heavy consumption of yeast products to see if a reaction occurs. The second purpose of a yeast-free diet is to reduce or eliminate sources of yeasty or moldy foods in one's diet and to minimize allergic reactions to these things.

—Dr. Sidney M. Baker, *Notes on the Yeast Problem*

As yeast-related illnesses have gained more popular attention, a number of treatment strategies have been proposed. One is the yeast-free diet described and explained in detail in a number of books on yeast-related illnesses like *The Missing Diagnosis, The Yeast Syndrome,* and *The Yeast Connection.* The diet has many variations but is based on the assumption that people who struggle with yeast as a medical condition are contributing to their health problems each time they consume yeast in food. The theory is that these people are hypersensitive to yeast to the extent that even the ingestion of small amounts of the organism or related organisms in foodstuffs (even if the yeasts are dead) triggers a disease response in the body.

The diet eliminates all yeast-containing foods—bread, most baked goods, beer, wine, liquor, and brewer's yeast. It also eliminates all foods that contain fungi (yeasts and molds are fungi)—all cheeses, mushrooms, and leftovers, for example. Additionally, you must avoid any food which is fermented, such as vinegar, soy sauce, mustard, mayonnaise, ketchup, and pickles. The diet also curtails the consumption of junk food or any food that is fried, refined, heavily processed, or loaded with sugar, salt, artificial additives, preservatives, or chemicals. For various reasons, the diet also eliminates coffee and tea (including herb tea), peanuts, smoked meats and fishes, dried fruit, all juices (except fresh squeezed), cheese-containing snacks, all foods which are breaded, buttermilk, sour cream, margarine. All fruits and vegetables must be peeled before eating. Finally, the diet restricts the ingestion of all carbohydrates (not just refined ones) since all carbohydrates break down into simple sugars in the digestive process. Some practitioners restrict carbohydrate intake to as low as 60 grams per day, the amount in one large bagel (56 grams) or one cup of chocolate pudding (67 grams).

Called the Yeast-Free Diet, the Candida Control Diet, or the Anticandida Diet, among other names, it is basically a regimen severely curtailing most foods other than fats and proteins, on which yeast cannot feed. Following the diet is made even more difficult by the prescription to avoid meat products from animals which were fed antibiotics, a common livestock industry practice in this country.

Advocates of this approach agree that the exact diet will vary for each individual, with trial and error playing an important role. They also agree that the restrictions can be eased as improvements in health are realized. However, the diet is a severe one and especially difficult to follow in restaurants and social situations or if individuals must maintain a special regimen (low cholesterol, kosher, or vegetarian regimes, for instance).

There is considerable controversy over the yeast-free diet. It would be almost impossible to accurately measure its success clinically due to the large number of uncontrollable variables. The exact requirements of the diet vary with each practitioner promoting it, and at this point, stories of its success are anecdotal. A large number of people who have attempted it felt it was too hard to follow long enough to see if it would make a real difference. Also, this kind of diet may have questionable long-term merit as high protein/low carbohydrate diets like it are generally considered to be unhealthy. Generally, it appears that people reporting the most success were those suffering from a number of maladies, of which recurrent yeast vaginitis was but one. Nor is it clear whether the improvements resulted from the avoidance of yeast or from other dietary changes made in the process.

Generally, a wholesome balanced diet filled with a variety of healthy foods is the most direct, long-term nutritional approach to treating infections. However, a short-term yeast-free diet may be worth trying. There is no good data on effectiveness, though some women report that yeasty vaginal discharge increases within a few hours of consuming foods they have identified as troublesome, with fruit most often implicated as the culprit.

The diet may be useful as a diagnostic tool, especially in medical conditions that recur with regularity. Dr. Baker, author of *Notes on the Yeast Problem,* suggests following the yeast-free diet strictly for a given period of time (from a minimum of five days up to several months), then to "challenge" the yeast by adding the previously restricted foods and observing the effect. If there is a reaction, he suggests repeating the procedure a number of times to narrow down the dietary culprits.

We ourselves at this stage do not recommend the yeast-free diet as a therapeutic regime for vaginal candidiasis. For further reading on yeast-related illnesses and the yeast-free diet, see Appendix C.

Guide to Taking Antibiotics

Every physician ordering antibiotics for the sexually active woman should be aware that many of these women will develop Candida vaginitis. This is not a threat to their lives, but the discomfort, inconvenience, and embarrassment of vaginal discharge and genital itching certainly reduce the quality of life. In addition, intercourse becomes a painful exercise to be avoided.

—Dr. William Ledger, *Infections in Medicine*

By adulthood, most people have taken dozens of courses of antibiotics, whether for acne, strep throat, ear infections, or other conditions. There is no question that antibiotics are truly miracle drugs; they literally save lives. Almost from their discovery only seven decades ago, antibiotics have saved lives and cured formerly deadly diseases, such as pneumonia, syphilis, and tuberculosis.

However, the limitations and potential dangers of these remarkable drugs are much less widely known. They are prescribed liberally, as if they were completely free of side effects. Yet we know that, in addition to creating a yeast overgrowth, they upset the gastrointestinal environment, often leading to digestive trouble, increased gas, and diarrhea, not to mention nausea, vomiting, and rashes. They can make you overly sensitive to sunlight and, in some people, cause allergic reactions, ranging from hives and vomiting to far more severe and occasionally life-threatening problems. They can trigger fever, jaundice, and even cause deafness. Also, taking antibiotics for conditions where they are not critical can result in the mutation of more resistant strains of bacteria in your body, so that you will then need stronger or different antibiotics to combat the same infection. The increase in strains of bacterial resistance to a particular antibiotic in fact is directly linked to inadequate dosage and inappropriate use of antibiotics.

There are a variety of potential organisms which cause disease. Antibiotics are only effective against bacteria, and don't work at all against viruses (the cause of, among other things, colds and flu) and parasites. Yet many people, ignorant of this, pressure their doctors to prescribe antibiotics for everything, and a number of physicians are willing to comply. Half of all patients who go to their doctors with colds, it has been estimated, receive an antibiotic which is useless. One study showed that 90 percent of penicillin usage was inappropriate. Surveys on hospital use of antibiotics show that 60 percent of the patients receive either an incorrect antibiotic, the wrong dosage, or a drug when none is required. This indiscriminate use is especially reprehensible when it complicates the correct diagnosis and appropriate treatment of a serious illness.

Antibiotics do not destroy all bacteria; they are generally classified as either broad spectrum or narrow spectrum. Narrow-spectrum antibiotics kill very specific bacteria, while broad-spectrum antibiotics are designed to kill a wide variety. Broad-spectrum antibiotics are simpler and easier for physicians to prescribe; there is no need to obtain a white blood cell count and bacterial culture to determine which narrow-spectrum ones will be effective. Unfortunately, the simplicity and ease of receiving broad-spectrum antibiotics is countered by the fact that they cause the most intestinal distress, irregular bowel function, and yeast infections when they wipe out the broad spectrum of helpful as well as harmful bacteria.

These are questions you should ask your doctor: Will a narrow spectrum one do the job and will the recommended antibiotic react with any other substances you use (large doses may impair the effectiveness of birth control pills)? Are eating times or drinking habits important? What side effects might occur? Antibiotics must be taken in the correct dosage and for the prescribed duration to be effective. Always take the full course even if your symptoms have disappeared; never take incomplete or leftover dosages or antibiotics prescribed for someone else.

You should always avoid using antibiotics whenever possible. When you have to use them, you can recognize and anticipate the risks—and avoid a resulting yeast infection!

Simultaneous antifungal therapy should be used as a preventative measure when you take these drugs if you are prone to yeast infections. Nystatin will prevent the development of thrush after antibiotic therapy, and using it concurrently with antibiotics will prevent an overgrowth of yeasts in the bowel. Ask your doctor for prescriptions for oral and intravaginal nystatin to cover the full course of the antibiotic therapy and for a few days after. Most doctors are aware of this problem and are more than willing to comply. If your doctor will not cooperate or you do not wish to take nystatin, a prescription for ACI-JEL (Ortho) should be requested. ACI-JEL, though costly, is an intravaginal acidic formulation that will maintain the correct pH in the vagina and dilute the yeast organisms trying to establish themselves. Without a prescription, you can use caprylic acid, Gyne-Lotrimin, Monistat 7, acidophilus, yogurt, and garlic as directed in chapter 5 to help counter the yeast-enhancing effects of antibiotic therapy.

Appendix B lists the drug and brand names of the major broad-spectrum and narrow-spectrum antibiotics to help you determine what kind you are taking.

The time is right for women to learn about the diseases that plague them and to arm themselves with the information they need to make informed and timely decisions. We hope this book will help serve that purpose. Please write to us with any comments or suggestions that you would like to share.

APPENDIX

A

GLOSSARY OF MEDICAL TERMS

Anorectal: refers to the anus and rectum.

Anus: the posterior opening of the alimentary canal (which consists of the mouth, pharynx, esophagus, stomach, small and large intestines, and serves the functions of digestion, absorption of food, and elimination of waste products).

Balanitis: an inflammation (with itchy discharge) of the glans penis, foreskin, and neighboring mucous membranes, often gonococcal.

Balanoposthitis: an inflammation of the glans penis and foreskin.

Commensal: one or two organisms that live in an intimate, nonparasitic relationship.

Cystitis: an inflammation of the bladder.

Distention: the state of being stretched out or inflated.

Dyspareunia: painful intercourse (from the Greek: "unhappily mated as bedfellows").

Endogenous: produced within a cell or organism.

Epithelial: the layer of cells forming the top surface of the skin and of the mucous and other membranes.

Excoriation: a raw, irritated lesion.

Fomites: objects which themselves are not infections, but are capable of transmitting infectious organisms, such as a wet towel or toothbrush.

Glans penis: the conical, bulbous end of the penis.

Introitus: any opening of the body, as in the external orifice of the vagina.

Mucus (also Mucous): a sticky, slippery secretion, produced by mucous membranes to moisten and protect the membranes.

Mycotic: an infection caused by fungus.

Parasite: a plant or animal that lives upon or within another living organism at whose expense it obtains some advantage.

Pathogen: any disease-producing microorganism or substance.

Prepuce: the foreskin of a penis.

Prophylactic medication: medicine given to prevent an illness, rather than to treat an illness.

Pruritus: severe itching.

Purulent: containing or consisting of pus.

Rectum: the end portion of the large intestine.

Speculum: an instrument inserted into the opening of the vagina, used to facilitate visual inspection or application of medication into the vagina.

Subclinical: the period before typical symptoms or signs of a disease appear.

Transudation: the passage of bodily fluids through a membrane or tissue surface; may or may not be the result of inflammation.

Ulceration: an abnormal break in the skin or mucous membrane, often associated with slow healing.

Urethra: the canal connecting the bladder to the outside opening of the body, running above the vaginal opening in women and through the penis in men.

Urethritis: an inflammation of the urethra.

Urticaria: an inflammatory reaction of the skin, associated with a sudden elevation of the skin surface and severe itching (wheal); can be induced by certain foods, drugs, infection, allergy, or stress.

Vaginitis: an inflammation of the vagina which becomes reddened and swollen, usually associated with a discharge.

Venereologist: a doctor who specializes in the treatment of venereal disease.

Vulva: the external parts of the female genitalia consisting of the labia majora, labia minora, clitoris, and vestibule.

Vulvae Pruritus: a disorder marked by severe itching of external female genitalia; often an early sign of diabetes.

Vulvitis: inflammation of the vulva, includes reddening, swelling, blistering, excoriation, and ulceration.

B

LIST OF BROAD-SPECTRUM AND NARROW-SPECTRUM ANTIBIOTICS

The following chart lists the names of the most common broad-spectrum and narrow-spectrum antibiotics. As discussed in chapters 2 and 6, antibiotic use can lead to yeast infections. Narrow-spectrum antibiotics kill fewer nonpathogenic bacteria than broad-spectrum antibiotics and therefore are preferable for women prone to yeast infections.

The names shown in capital letters are the drug names; the names listed under them are some of the many brand names under which the drugs are sold.

PARTIAL LISTING OF ANTIBIOTICS

NARROW-SPECTRUM ANTIBIOTICS	BROAD-SPECTRUM ANTIBIOTICS
ERYTHROMYCIN	**AMOXICILLIN**
Bristamycin	Amoxil
E-Mycin	Augmentin
Eramycin	Larotid
Eryc	Novamoxin

NARROW-SPECTRUM ANTIBIOTICS

Erypar
EryPed
Ery-Tab
Ethril
Ilosone
Ilotycin
Pediamycin
Pfizer-E
Wyamycin

PENICILLIN G

Bicillin
Crystapen
Crysticillin
Duracillin
Megacillin
Penioral
Pentids
Permapen
Pfizerpen G
Staphcillin
Wycillin

PENICILLIN V

Beepen VK
Betapen-VK
Compocillin VK
Ledercillin VK
Novapen V
Pen-V
Pen-Vee K
Penapar VK
Pfizerpen VK
Robicillin VK
Suspen

BROAD-SPECTRUM ANTIBIOTICS

Penamox
Polymox
Robamox
Utimox
Wymox

AMPICILLIN

Alpen
Amcill
Ampicin
Cyclacillin
Omnipen
Penbritin
Polycillin
Principen
SK-Ampillin
Supen
Totacillin

CEPHALOSPORIN

Anspor
Ceclor
Ceporex
Duricef
Keflex
Novolexin
Ultracef
Velosef

CHLORAMPHENICOL

Amphicol
Antibiopto
Chloromycetin
Chloroptic
Econochlor

NARROW-SPECTRUM ANTIBIOTICS

Uticillin VK
V-Cillin K
Veetids

BROAD-SPECTRUM ANTIBIOTICS

Mychel
Novochlorocap
Ophthochlor
Pentamycetin

TETRACYCLINE

Achromycin
Achrostatin V
Bio-Tetra
Bristacycline
Cyclopar
Medicycline
Neo-Tetrine
Novotetra
Panmycin
Retet
Robitet
SK-Tetracycline
Tetrachel
Tetracyn
Tetracyrine
Tetrastatin
Tetrex

C

SUGGESTED READING

Women's Health

The Complete Guide to Women's Health by B. Shepard and C. Shepard, Plume, 1990, $14.95

The Medical SelfCare Book of Women's Health by B. Hasselbring, S. Greenwood, and M. Castleman, Doubleday & Co., 1987, $12.95

The New Our Bodies, OurSelves by the Boston Women's Health Collective, Simon & Schuster, 1984, $12.95

My Body, My Health: The Concerned Women's Book of Gynecology by F. Stewart, F. Guest, G. Stewart, and R. Hatcher, Bantam Books, 1981, $9.95

Every Woman's Book by P. Airola, Health Plus, 1979, $17.95

Yeast-Related Illnesses

The Yeast Connection by W. Crook, Professional Books, 1989, $8.95

The Yeast Syndrome by J. Trowbridge and M. Walker, Bantam Books, 1986, $3.95

The Missing Diagnosis by C. O. Truss, The Missing Diagnosis, Inc., 1985, $8.95

Candida Albicans: Can Yeast Be Your Problem by L. Chaitow, Thorsons, 1987, $4.95

Understanding Candida by P. de Ruyter, Prism Books, 1989, $8.95

Food Allergies

Is This Your Child: Discovering and Treating Unrecognized Allergies by D. Rapp, William Morrow, 1991, $19.95

Hidden Food Allergies: How to discover if you have food allergies and what to do to successfully overcome them by S. H. Astor, Avery Publishing Group, 1988, $7.95

Brain Allergies by N. Orenstein, Publishers Group West, 1987, $12.95

Allergies and Your Family by D. Rapp, Sterling, 1980, $12.95

THE FDA HEARINGS: JUNE 1990

•

> Vaginal candidiasis . . . is a self-limited and usually benign condition.
>
> —Dr. Douglass Given, Schering-Plough, makers of Gyne-Lotrimin

> I have heard a lot of talk about the self-limiting nature of Candida vaginitis, but I think that severe forms of Candida vaginitis are as self-limiting as being hit by a truck.
>
> —Dr. Jack Sobel, Wayne State University

Yeast infections have been around since time immemorial, but beginning in the late 1980s, a new burst of attention by drug companies, the FDA, and the media has brought discussion of these infections to the public eye. Over the second half of the decade, a number of new antiyeast infection products were introduced, sold largely through health food stores. In 1988

Schering-Plough, makers of Gyne-Lotrimin vaginal cream and suppositories, petitioned the Food and Drug Administration (FDA) to reclassify their prescription antifungal formulations as over-the-counter (OTC) remedies. This push was motivated by the fact that the patents were about to expire on several of the long-standing prescription preparations. These events expanded the potential market for antiyeast remedies, and the rush to "educate" women about self-diagnosis and treatment for yeast infections was on.

Schering-Plough received final permission from the FDA in November 1990 to begin selling its products without prescription. Johnson and Johnson, makers of Monistat 7 cream and suppositories through its Ortho Pharmaceuticals unit, in the meantime also decided to join in the reclassification effort. They, too, received an FDA go-ahead, with final permission granted in February 1991. The two companies are expected to spend as much as $100 million to woo women to buy their products. Promotional activities are planned for consumer magazines, network television, doctors' waiting rooms, and even high school health classes. For instance, Schering-Plough is conducting a huge marketing effort through their education of women about vaginal illness. Their activities include the distribution of a free video, *What Every Woman Should Know: Vaginal Yeast Infections*, to high schools, teaching modules for health classes, and manuals for nurse practitioners on educating women in self-diagnosis.

The move initiated by Schering-Plough to reclassify the medications was not the first time the reclassification issue had come up at the FDA. Ten years ago, the FDA reviewed the prescription antifungals to determine if any of them should be recategorized as OTCs. They consulted with a group of military doctors who determined that antifungals sold for athlete's foot and jock itch (male problems) could be reclassified while those (identical) antifungals sold for vaginal yeast infections should remain prescription drugs.

In 1982 Schering-Plough sought nonprescription status for Gyne-Lotrimin for the first time. The FDA refused to consider their petition, saying it was concerned that women wouldn't be able to properly diagnose themselves. In 1988 Schering-Plough again petitioned the FDA to alter the status of their Gyne-Lotrimin (clotrimazole) products. The FDA again turned down their application, which was, however, revived by an FDA advisory committee which said that, within certain guidelines, there were valid reasons to increase access to the drugs.

Now, more than a decade after athlete's foot formulations were made OTC, "female" antifungals are finally achieving the same status as "male" antifungals.

The FDA is not a proactive organization. It responds to petitions brought to it. This is invariably done by drug companies who anticipate a financial gain in securing a favorable ruling to its petitions. There is almost always a financial incentive involved, although this is not always the case, as in the efforts of AIDS activists who secured wider distribution of AZT.

Federal regulations provide for the switching of a prescription drug to OTC use when the commissioner finds that such requirements are not necessary for the protection of the public health by reason of the drug's toxicity, other potentiality for harmful effect, the method of its use, or the collateral measures necessary to its use, and when the commissioner finds that the drug is safe and effective for use in self-medication as directed in the proposed labeling.

Ironically, the FDA does not review a drug, per se, it reviews an application for a specific product from a specific company. So even though Gyne-Lotrimin and Monistat 7 ultimately received approval, that does not translate into blanket approval of other preparations made from the same drugs in the same strength for the same condition. This has resulted in a dichotomy of drugs—those antifungals that can now be purchased OTC and those antifungals that must be purchased by prescription—even though there is significant overlap in those two categories. While this is a bit crazy, it does offer some advantages. Women with health insurance can buy the preparations as prescriptions and receive whatever discounts their insurance companies pay, while women who do not have insurance or chose not to use it, can walk into any drugstore and walk out with their medication.

Notably, these are the first OTC drugs approved to treat vaginal yeast infections. All the other OTC remedies available cannot say on their labels that they are for the treatment of yeast infections; they can only say they relieve itching, irritation, discharge, etc. The FDA cited as main reasons in awarding the reclassification the long history of safety for these products as well as the minimal harm that could befall consumers in using these products on a misdiagnosed infection.

The FDA has essentially never allowed an OTC product to use the word *cure* in its labeling. Over-the-counter drugs are not supposed to *cure* things, rather, they are supposed to be mild forms of drugs geared to providing short-term relief from minor discomforts. Both Gyne-Lotrimin and Monistat, with the FDA's blessing, claim to "cure" yeast infections. This is ironic because the products have been around for almost 20 years, during which time recurrence has been a big problem.

The recognition that women can diagnose themselves and have available more treatment options is laudable. But yeast infections are still an issue and cure is still an unmet goal for many women. These antifungal prescriptions, available both in drugstores and pharmacies, are one more tool women can use to eradicate their painful, messy infections.

These antifungals are also big business. In 1990, the last year these drugs were prescription items, the total market for prescription antiyeast vaginal medications was $220 million. Schering-Plough and Johnson and Johnson will sell $150 million of their OTC versions in their first year alone—more than double original estimates. Sales of OTC yeast medications are expected to top $400 million by 1995.

The efforts of Schering-Plough and the FDA to bring these drugs directly to the consumer benefits women. But what would benefit women more is additional research into the causes and long-term cures for recurrent yeast vaginitis.

REFERENCES AND NOTES

Introduction

Page 1: M. Leegaard, "The Incidence of *Candida Albicans* in the Vagina of 'Healthy Young Women,'" *Acta Obstet Gynecol Scand*, 63 (1984).

Page 2: J. D. Sobel, "Recurrent Vulvovaginal Candidiasis," *New England Journal of Medicine*, vol. 315, no. 23 (1986).

Page 2: J. P. Trowbridge and M. Walker, *The Yeast Syndrome* (New York: Bantam Books, 1986).

Chapter One

Page 31: A. L. Hilton and D. W. Warnock, "Vaginal Candidiasis and the Role of the Digestive Tract as a Source of Infection," *British Journal of Obstetrics and Gynaecology*, vol. 82 (November 1975).

Chapter Two

Page 35: F. Davidson and R. F. Mould, "Recurrent Genital Candidosis in Women and the Effects of Intermittent Prophylactic Treatment," *British Journal of Venereal Diseases* (1978).

Page 38: J. W. Rippon, *Medical Mycology, The Pathogenic Fungi and the Pathogenic Actinomycetes* (Philadelphia: W. B. Saunders Company, 1974).

Page 44: R. S. Morton and S. Rashid, "Candidal Vaginitis: Natural History, Predisposing Factors and Prevention," Proceedings of the Royal Society of Medicine, 70 [Supplement 4] (1977).

Page 45: G. R. G. Monif, "Classification and Pathogenesis of Vulvovaginal Candidiasis," (Proceedings from the International Symposium on Vulvovaginal Mycoses), *American Journal of Obstetrics and Gynecology*, vol. 152, no. 7 (August 1985).

Page 45: R. Lopez-Martinez et al, "Vaginal Candidosis," *Mycopathologia* 85 (1984).

Page 45: P. J. H. Tooley, "Patient and Doctor Preferences in the Treatment of Vaginal Candidosis," *The Practitioner*, vol. 229 (1985).

Page 46: I. Milsom and L. Forssman, "Repeated Candidiasis: Reinfection or Recrudescence?" (A review. Proceedings from the International Symposium on Vulvovaginal Mycoses), *American Journal of Obstetrics and Gynecology*, vol. 152, no. 7 (August 1985).

Page 49: R. Hurley, "Trends in Candidal Vaginitis," Proceedings of the Royal Society of Medicine, 70 [Supplement 4] (1977).

Page 54: R. Lopez-Martinez, D. Ruiz-Sanchez, and E. Vertiz-Chavez, "Vaginal Candidosis," *Mycopathologia* 85 (1984).

Pages 52–53: R. C. Wunderlich, Jr., and D. K. Kalita, "*Candida Albicans:* How to Fight an Exploding Epidemic of Yeast-Related Diseases," (Keats Publishing, New Canaan, CT, 1984).

Page 55: R. N. Thin, M. Leighton, and M. J. Dixon, "How Often Is Genital Yeast Infection Sexually Transmitted," *British Medical Journal* (July 1977).

Page 55: J. D. Sobel, "Epidemiology and Pathogenesis of Recurrent Vulvovaginal Candidiasis," (Proceedings from the

International Symposium on Vulvovaginal Mycoses), *American Journal of Obstetrics and Gynecology,* vol. 152, no. 7 (August 1985).

Page 58: J. M. Merkus, M. P. Bisschop, and L. A. M. Stolte, "The Proper Nature of Vaginal Candidiosis and the Problem of Recurrence," *Obstetrical and Gynecological Survey,* 40 (1985).

Page 61: M. J. Rosenberg, W. Roganapithayakorn, P. J. Feldblum and J. E. Higgins, "Effect of the Contraceptive Sponge on Chlamydial Infection, Gonorrhea, and Candidiasis," *Journal of the American Medical Association,* vol. 257, no. 17 (May 1, 1987).

Page 62: H. I. Winner and R. Hurley, *Candida Albicans,* (Boston: Little, Brown and Company, 1964).

Pages 64–65: B. J. Horowitz, S. W. Edelstein, and L. Lippman, "Sugar Chromatography Studies in Recurrent Candida Vulvovaginitis, *Journal of Reproductive Medicine,* vol. 29 (1984).

Page 66: H. I. Winner and R. Hurley, *Candida Albicans,* (Boston: Little, Brown and Company, 1964).

Chapter Three

Page 70: L. Chaitow, *"Candida Albicans,* Could Yeast Be Your Problem?" (Rochester, VT: Thornsons Publishers, 1987).

Page 72: F. C. Odds, *Candida and Candidosis,* (Baltimore: University Park Press, 1979).

Page 72: R. D. Catterall, "Influence of Gestogenic Contraceptive Pills on Vaginal Candidosis," *British Journal of Venereal Disease,* 47 (1971).

Page 74: R. N. Thin, M. Leighton, and M. J. Dixon, "How Often Is Genital Yeast Infection Sexually Transmitted," *British Medical Journal* (July 1977).

Page 74: J. D. Sobel, "Epidemiology and Pathogenesis of Recurrent Vulvovaginal Candidiasis," (Proceedings from the International Symposium on Vulvovaginal Mycoses), *Amer-*

ican Journal of Obstetrics and Gynecology, vol. 152, no. 7 (August 1985).

Page 74: T. E. Drake and H. I. Maibach, "Candida and Candidiasis," *Postgraduate Medicine* 53, no. 3 (March 1973).

Page 77: M. Leegaard, "The Incidence of *Candida Albicans* in the Vagina of 'Healthy Young Women,'" *Acta Obstet Gynecol Scand,* 63 (1984).

Page 81: Discussion from the Proceedings from the International Symposium on Vulvovaginal Mycoses, *American Journal of Obstetrics and Gynecology,* vol. 152, no. 7 (August 1985).

Page 81: J. D. Sobel, "Vulvovaginal Candidiasis—What We Know and Do Not Know," *Annals of Internal Medicine,* vol. 101, no. 3 (1984).

Page 82: J. W. Rippon, *Medical Mycology, the Pathogenic Fungi and the Pathogenic Actinomycetes,* (Philadelphia: W. B. Saunders Company, 1974).

Page 84: A. L. Hilton and D. W. Warnock, "Vaginal Candidiasis and the Role of the Digestive Tract as a Source of Infection," *British Journal of Obstetrics and Gynaecology,* vol. 82 (November 1975).

Page 84: J. D. Oriel, "Clinical Overview of Candidal Vaginitis," Proceedings of the Royal Society of Medicine, vol. 70, (1977).

Page 84: J. D. Sobel, "Epidemiology and Pathogenesis of Recurrent Vulvovaginal Candidiasis," (Proceedings from the International Symposium on Vulvovaginal Mycoses), *American Journal of Obstetrics and Gynecology,* vol. 152, no. 7 (August 1985).

Pages 84–85: H. I. Winner and R. Hurley *Candida Albicans,* (Boston: Little, Brown and Company, 1964).

Page 86: J. W. Rippon, *Medical Mycology, the Pathogenic Fungi and the Pathogenic Actinomycetes,* (Philadelphia: W. B. Saunders Company, 1974).

Page 95: G. R. G. Monif, "Classification and Pathogenesis of Vulvovaginal Candidiasis," (Proceedings from the International Symposium on Vulvovaginal Mycoses), *American*

Journal of Obstetrics and Gynecology, vol. 152, no. 7 (August 1985).

Page 100: F. Fleury, "Adult Vaginitis," *Clinical Obstetrics and Gynecology,* vol. 24, no. 2 (June 1981).

Page 102: L. J. Cibley, "Vulvovaginitis: Current Approach to Diagnosis and Treatment," *The Female Patient,* vol. 11 (February 1986).

Page 106: J. E. Bennett, "Searching for the Yeast Connection," *The New England Journal of Medicine,* vol. 323, no. 25 (December 1990).

Page 107: W. E. Dismukes, J. S. Wade, J. Y. Lee, B. K. Dockery and J. D. Hain, "Randomized Double-Blind Trial of Nystatin Therapy for the Candidiasis Hypersensitivity Syndrome," *The New England Journal of Medicine,* vol. 323, no. 25 (December 1990).

Page 107: L. Chaitow, *"Candida Albicans:* Could Yeast Be Your Problem?" (Rochester, VT: Thornsons Publishers, 1987).

Chapter Four

Page 110: J. D. Sobel, "Vulvovaginal Candidiasis—What We Know and Do Not Know," *Annals of Internal Medicine,* vol. 101, no. 3 (1984).

Page 111: P. J. H. Tooley, "Patient and Doctor Preferences in the Treatment of Vaginal Candidosis," *The Practitioner,* vol. 229 (1985).

Page 117: R. S. Morton, Discussion from Trends in Candidal Vaginitis Meeting (Proceedings of the Royal Society of Medicine, 70 [Supplement 4] (1977).

Page 118: Interview with Dr. Jack Sobel, Detroit, MI, January 1987.

Page 128: R. Hurley, "Inveterate Vaginal Thrush," *The Practitioner* (December 1975).

Chapter Five

Page 133: S. M. Baker, "Notes on the Yeast Problem" (New Haven, CT: Gesell Institute of Human Development, 1985).

Page 141: A. Friedlander, M. M. Druker, and A. Schachter, "Lactobacillus Acidophilus and Vitamin B Complex in the Treatment of Vaginal Infection," *Panminerva Medica*, 28 (1986).

Page 144: A. L. Hilton and D. W. Warnock, "Vaginal Candidiasis and the Role of the Digestive Tract as a Source of Infection," *British Journal of Obstetrics and Gynaecology*, vol. 82 (November 1975).

Page 145: Investigators studying the mode of infection in candidal vulvovaginitis have found that the incidence of this condition was much higher in patients harboring yeasts in the intestinal tract. Miles, et al, (M. R. Miles, L. Olsen, A. Rogers, "Recurrent Vaginal Candidiasis," *Journal of the American Medical Association*, 238: 1836–1837, no. 17, October 24, 1977) found that in women with recurrent vaginal candidiasis, there was a 100 percent association between the presence of *C. albicans* in the feces and in the vagina. Another study found that over 70 percent of patients with vaginal infection harbor the same Candida species in the vagina as in the ano-rectal tract. Dissemination of yeasts from the gastrointestinal tract may be more widespread than had previously been thought.

Page 146: G. J. Dennerstein and R. Langley, "Vulvovaginal Candidiasis: Treatment and Recurrence," *Australian/New Zealand Journal of Obstetrics and Gynaecology*, 22 (1982).

Page 157: K. D. Gunston and P. F. Fairbrother, "Treatment of Vaginal Discharge with Yoghurt," *South Africa Medical Journal* (April 1975).

Page 158: A. Pike, "Garlic's Natural Medicinal Qualities," *Let's Live* (November 1990).

Page 160: T. E. Swate and J. C. Weed, "Boric Acid

Treatment of Vulvovaginal Candidiasis," *Obstetrics and Gynecology,* vol. 43, no. 6 (June 1974).

Page 161: American Journal of Obstetrics and Gynecology (1981), cited in *WomenWise,* "Remedy for Vaginal Yeast Infection: Boric Acid Powder," vol. 5, no. 1 (Spring 1982).

Page 172: F. C. Odds, "Cure and Relapse with Antifungal Therapy," Proceedings of the Royal Society of Medicine, vol. 70, (1977).

Page 181: F. Fleury, "Adult Vaginitis," *Clinical Obstetrics and Gynecology,* vol. 24, no. 2 (June 1981).

Page 189: C. O. Truss, *The Missing Diagnosis* (Birmingham, AL: The Missing Diagnosis, Inc., 1985).

Page 188: J. N. Henderson and I. B. Tait, "The Use of Povidone-Iodine ('Betadine') Pessaries in the Treatment of Candidal and Trichomonal Vaginitis," *Current Medical Research and Opinion,* vol. 3, no. 3 (1975).

Page 189: J. N. Henderson and I. B. Tait, "The Use of Povidone-Iodine ('Betadine') Pessaries in the Treatment of Candidal and Trichomonal Vaginitis," *Current Medical Research and Opinion,* vol. 3, no. 3 (1975).

Page 191: R. S. Morton and S. Rashid, "Candidal Vaginitis: Natural History, Predisposing Factors and Prevention," Proceedings of the Royal Society of Medicine, 70 [Supplement 4] (1977).

Page 191: R. N. Thin, M. Leighton, and M. J. Dixon, "How Often Is Genital Yeast Infection Sexually Transmitted," *British Medical Journal* (July 1977).

Page 192: J. D. Sobel, "Epidemiology and Pathogenesis of Recurrent Vulvovaginal Candidiasis," (Proceedings from the International Symposium on Vulvovaginal Mycoses), *American Journal of Obstetrics and Gynecology,* vol. 152, no. 7 (August 1985).

Page 199: D. McNellis, M. McLeod, J. Lawson, and S. A. Pasquale, "Treatment of Vulvovaginal Candidiasis in Pregnancy: A Comparative Study," *Obstetrics and Gynecology,* vol. 50, no. 6 (December 1977).

Page 209: G. J. Dennerstein, "Depo-Provera in the Treatment of Recurrent Vulvovaginal Candidiasis," *The Journal of Reproductive Medicine,* vol. 31, no. 9 (September 1986).

Chapter Six

Page 221: S. M. Baker, "Notes on the Yeast Problem" (New Haven, CT: Gesell Institute of Human Development, 1985).

Page 229: S. Rashid, M. Collins, J. Corner, and R. S. Morton, "Survival of *Candida Albicans* on Fabric After Laundering," *British Journal of Venereal Disease,* 60 (4) 277 (1984).

Page 230: M. Leegaard, "The Incidence of *Candida Albicans* in the Vagina of 'Healthy Young Women,'" *Acta Obstet Gynecol Scand,* 63 (1984).

Page 237: W. Ledger, "Editorial Comment on Defective Immune Responses in Patients with Recurrent Candidiasis," by S. S. Witkin, *Infections in Medicine,* (May/June 1985).

Note to readers: The reference list appearing above is a partial listing of the materials used for the research and compilation of this book. A full listing of the resource documents can be obtained by writing to the authors.

INDEX

t = table, *f* = figure

A & D (ointment), 204
Abrasions/irritations, 12, 39,
  51, 52, 60–62, 227–28
Acidity (vagina), *see* pH
Acidophilus, 69, 138–42, 155,
  203–04, 239
  use during pregnancy, 198,
  199
ACI-JEL, 155–56, 239
Acyclovir (Zovirax), 100
Addiction(s), 219, 220, 224
Age, 1, 7, 87, 103, 205, 206
AIDS, 33, 101, 103, 126, 208,
  225
Alcohol, 25–26, 213, 219–20
Alkalinity (vagina), *see* pH
Allergic reactions, 183, 184–90
  to douches, 170
  in sexual partners, 192–93
Allergies, 57, 96, 105
  food, 203, 218
Aloe vera, 152, 166–67
Alternative therapies, 3, 4, 150
Anal sex, 53, 58–60, 98
Antiboiotic therapy, 1
  in children, 68–69
  full course of, 104
  as predisposing condition, 34,
    39, 40–44, 106, 121, 136
Antibiotics, 6, 15, 30, 87, 89,
  112, 134, 212

broad/narrow-spectrum, 137,
  212, 238–40, 244–46
guide to taking, 237–40
indiscriminate use of, 238
ingested with food, 42–44,
  235
prevention of yeast infections
  when using, 188
and sugar cravings, 216
in treatment of chlamydia, 97
in treatment of gardnerella,
  96
in treatment of gonorrhea, 98
upsetting yeast/bacteria ratio,
  137, 142
use of, and rise in yeast infections, 11–12
Antibody tests, 96–97
Anticandida Diet, 235
Antifungal therapy, 13, 69, 72,
  96, 172–83
  courses of, 144
  during pregnancy, 199
  in prevention of yeast infec-
    tions, 96, 97, 98, 239
Antifungals, 10, 12, 15, 46, 82,
  118, 141, 143, 149, 172–
  83
  broad-spectrum, 179, 182
  costs of, 176–77*t*
  with diaphragm, 231

263

Antifungals (*cont.*)
efficacy of, 14
garlic as, 159
intravaginal, 42, 120, 121
new, 208
nondrug, 149, 150, 183–91
oral contraceptives and, 225
oral/topical, 67, 94, 108, 145–46, 152, 172–73, 195, 206
primary cure rate, 13
reclassified to over-the-counter, 250–51, 252–53
in treatment of sexual partner(s), 195
Anus, 5, 145, 152, 195, 201, 229
hygiene, 228, 229
transmission of yeasts from, 58, 59, 231
Athlete's foot, 33, 36, 105, 159, 166, 174, 182, 204, 250, 251

Bacterial infections, 30, 36, 95, 97
Bacterium(a), 31, 89, 96
beneficial, 16, 41, 69, 179
manipulation of, 209–10
resistant strains of, 237–38
yeast-controlling, 137–43
see also Lactobacilli
Bathing, 230
Betadine, 189
Biochemical individuality, 214
Birth canal, 1, 31, 68, 100
Birth control, 55, 87, 103, 112, 134, 225–26, 228, 230
see also Oral contraceptives
Blood, 6, 48, 51, 231
Blood sugar levels, 219
Body
chemical makeup of, 12
fuel for, 214–21
yeast-fighting defenses, 17
see also Healthy body
Boric acid, 152, 160–62

Boric acid ointment, 145, 161–62, 195
Borofax, 161
Bowel, 33, 58, 178
Breast-feeding, 33, 81, 101
as predisposing condition, 39, 49–52
treatment during, 149, 151, 179, 187, 199
Burows solution, 152, 166
Butoconazole, 172, 179, 181

Caffeine, 219–20
Calendula cream, 152, 167–69, 203, 204
Candida (genus), 31
Candida albicans, 1, 7, 8, 10–11, 31–33, 76, 90, 95, 116, 221
as indication of infection, 83–84
opportunistic, 38, 39
organisms of, 117*f*
pathogenic, 32, 33
significance of, 33–34
Candida balanitis, 56, 193
Candida balanoposthitis, 56, 193
Candida Control Diet, 235
Candida infections, 32
see also Vaginal yeast infections
Candidal vaginitis, 53
Candidal vulvovaginitis, 1
Candidiasis/Candidosis, 7, 31, 37–38, 83
incidence of, 41
see also Vaginal yeast infections
Candidosis, 7, 83
Caprylic acid, 108, 145, 147, 184, 186–88, 195, 239
Caprystatin, 187
Carbohydrates, refined, 64–65

Carriers, asymptomatic, 57, 96, 192
Cervical cancer, 101, 113–16
Cervicitis, 101–2
Chemical irritation, 61, 230
Chemical sensitivity, 105, 106
Childbirth as predisposing condition, 39, 49–52, 61
Children, 42, 181
    see also Infants
Chlamydia, 61, 93, 96–97, 209
Chlamydia test, 116
Chronic candidiasis, *see* Vaginal yeast infections
Cleanliness, 196, 198
    see also Hygiene
Clothing, 211, 229, 232–33
Clotrimazole, 172, 173, 179, 180–81, 251
Condoms, 94, 103, 104, 180, 195, 226, 228, 230
Contraception, *see* Birth control; Oral contraceptives
Contraceptive sponge, 61, 89, 225, 226, 227
Corticosteriods, 62–63
Cortisone, 63, 136, 204
Costs, 3, 4, 14
    emotional, 4, 14, 16, 88, 123–30
    of medications, 176–77*t*, 185
Creams, 2, 82, 204
    antifungal, 172, 173, 195
    imidazoles, 180, 181
Cure, 252
    four-point strategy for, 133–49
    spontaneous, 37
Cure rate(s), 13, 14, 144, 160, 172, 181, 188
    during pregnancy, 196, 199

Debilitation, 38, 39–40, 60, 191
Denture-wearers, 60–61, 205, 206

Deodorant preparations, 61
Desenex, 204, 206
Desitin, 204
Diabetes, 80–81, 89
Diagnosis, 117–20
    incorrect, 153, 182, 195
    need for correct, 104, 110–11, 151
    see also Self-diagnosis
Diaper rash, 33, 67, 73, 105, 178, 201–5
Diapers, sterilizing, 67, 191, 202, 229–30
Diaphragm, 61, 89, 180, 225, 226, 227, 228
    hygiene and, 229
    for menstruation, 231
Diet, 48, 64–65, 66, 106, 134, 213, 214–21
    ingesting antibiotics through, 42–44
    for nursing mothers, 52
    poor, 89
    in prevention, 211
    in pregnancy, 51
    in treatment of PSCC, 108
    see also Nutrition; Yeast-Free Diet
Digestive disturbances, 137–38
Discharge, vaginal, 1, 2, 10, 49–50, 88, 113, 134, 232
    acidophilus in treatment of, 141
    conditions causing unusual, 92–100
    diet and, 236
    douching and, 169, 170
    examining in wet mount, 116
    normal, 87–88, 226
    odor, 90, 92, 93, 95, 209
    during pregnancy, 197–98
    type and amount of, 87, 88, 89
    white, cheesy, 51, 90, 92, 196
    yeast load in, 86

Disease(s)
  Candida in, 32
  germ theory of, 29
Disease-fighting ability, impaired, 212
  see also Immune system
Doctors, 2–4, 123, 124–25, 198
  and diagnosis of vaginal yeast infections, 118–19, 120
  homeopathic, 162
  and treatment during pregnancy, 198–99
Doderlein cytolysis, 102
Douche bags, 170, 229
Douches, douching, 12, 61, 89, 113, 141, 169–71
  aloe vera, 167
  boric acid, 160, 161
  gentian violet, 190
  mouthwashes, 60
  povidone-iodine, 96, 189
  during pregnancy, 199
  in prevention, 227
  rules for, 171
  vinegar, 94, 103, 152–53, 154–55, 231
  yogurt, 142, 156, 157
Drug efficacy information, 14
Drugs, 12, 87, 220
  see also Prescription drugs

Ecological Formulas (co.), 59, 187, 188, 206
Emotional costs, 4, 14, 16, 88, 123–30
Endometritis, 93
Ergot, 30
Esophagus, inflamed, 33
Estrogen, 45, 47, 50–51, 56, 101, 197
Estrogen replacement, 6, 209
Exercise, 213, 222–23

Fatigue, 48, 49, 76, 105, 187, 224
Femicine, 165
Feminine hygiene sprays, 230
Fermentation, 25–26, 28, 29, 216
Fertility, 102, 110
Fetus, 31
Food, 33, 215–16
  see also Diet; Nutrition
Food allergies, 203, 218
Food and Drug Administration, 163, 184, 249–53
Fungal disease, 9, 10, 32
  immunity to, 36–37
Fungal infections, 33–34, 54, 64, 106, 182
Fungicides, *see* antifungal
Fungus(i), 8, 16, 21–34, 89, 108, 138, 145
  eliminating from diet, 234
  resistant strains of, 179
  species of, 23

Gardnerella, 90, 91
Gardnerella vaginitis (Hemophilus), 95–96
Garlic, 152, 158–60, 199, 239
Gastrointestinal tract, 186, 187
  reducing yeast in, 144–51
  yeasts in, 31, 58
Genepax, 190
Generic drugs, 204, 207
Genital abrasions/irritations, 38, 51, 52, 60–62, 136
  see also Abrasions/irritations
Genital infections, 7, 58, 193
Genital transmission, 73
  see also Sexual transmission
Gentian violet, 184, 190–91, 199, 206–07
Germ theory of disease, 29
Glucose, 25, 46, 138
Glucose tolerance test, 80–81

Glycogen, 50–51
Gonorrhea, 10, 61, 93, 96, 97–98, 126, 209, 225
Gonorrhea culture, 116
Gynecological care, 123
Gyne-Lotrimin, 135f, 165, 173, 175, 204, 206, 239, 250–53

Health, 17, 211–13
  compromised, 38–39
  exercise and, 222–23
  during pregnancy, 51
  strengthening, 135–37
Health insurance, 185, 252
Healthy body, 36, 59, 69
  natural immunity, 62
  resistance to fungi, 34
  yeast in, 32, 84
Hemophilus, 95–96
Herpes, 98–101, 123, 126
Herxheimer reaction, 147, 187
HIV positive, 64
  see also AIDS
Home remedies, 12, 92, 104, 122, 143, 149–50, 151–71, 181, 184–85, 211–12
  see also alternative therapies
  combining, 169
  gardnerella vaginitis, 96
  use during pregnancy, 199
  for symptomatic relief, 168t
  in treatment of diaper rash, 203–4
  trichomonas vaginitis, 94
Home testing kits, 81, 208–09
Homeopathic medicine, 152, 162–65, 199
Hormonal changes, 45, 47–48, 49, 197, 231–32
Hormonal manipulation, 209
Hormones, 5–6, 12, 87
Hygiene, 12, 211, 227, 228–30
  for sexual partners, 193

Hypersensitivity, yeast, 105, 107, 108, 234

Illness, 89
  as predisposing condition, 39, 40, 64–66, 135–36
  underlying, 38, 41
  see also Disease; Underlying condition
Imidazoles, 82, 172, 174t, 179–82
Immune system, 30, 33, 159, 164
  immature, 66–67, 200, 206
  weakness in, as predisposing condition, 40, 64–66, 136, 208
Immunity
  to fungal diseases, 36–37
  suppression of, 62–63
Immunology, 29
Immunosuppressant therapy
  as predisposing condition, 34, 39, 62–63, 121
Immunosuppressants, 6, 12, 112
Infancy, 66–69
Infantile thrush, 191
  see also Oral thrush
Infants, 9, 96, 100, 200–01
  exposure to yeast, 31–32
  yeast infections in, 1, 149
  see also Children
Infection/reinfection cycle, see Recurrence
Intercourse, 53–58, 59, 61, 89, 103, 104
  avoiding, 97, 99, 103, 113
  painful, 14, 90, 92, 93, 101, 122
  during treatment, 195
Intermittent Prophylactic Therapy (IPT), 82
Interpersonal relations, 123, 125–27, 128

Intestines, 33, 137–38,
    178
  yeast organisms in, 144–51
Itching, 1, 88, 90, 92, 134, 141
  with herpes, 98, 99
  see also Jock itch

Jock itch, 5, 33, 250
Johnson and Johnson (co.), 175,
    250

Ketoconazole, 57, 150, 172,
    179, 182–83, 199
K-Y Jelly, 61, 228

Lactobacilli, 102, 137–43, 153,
    226
  in yogurt, 156, 157
Lactobacilli vaccines, 209–10
"Law of similars," 162
Leisure time, 211
Lesbian sex, 53, 58–60, 196
Lesbians, 1, 123
Lifestyle, 65, 105, 212, 213–14
Liver, 33, 183
L-Lysine, 100
Lubricants, vaginal, 52, 61, 101
Lubrication, 61, 89, 228
Lysergic acid, 30

Malnutrition, 6
  see also Nutrition
Marigold Ointment, *see* Calen-
    dula cream
Medical approach/model, 38,
    117–23, 125, 128, 143,
    184
Medical care, 213
  nontraditional, 122
  when and why to seek, 16
Medical conditions associated
    with yeast, 71, 104–8

Medical history, 110, 112
Medical mycology, 33–34
Men, 5
  asymptomatic carriers, 57–58
  Candida in, 54
  role in women's yeast infec-
    tions, 55–56
  symptoms of chlamydia, 96
  uncircumcised, 54, 74, 192,
    193
  see also Sexual transmission
Menopause, 92, 101, 112, 209
Menstrual management, 230–32
  as predisposing condition, 39,
    47–49
Menstruation, 82, 87, 94, 101,
    103, 212
  and pH, 227
  treatment during, 179, 180
  and yeast, 75–76, 136
Metronidazole (Flagyl), 94, 96
Miconazole, 146, 172, 174, 179,
    181, 199
  see also Imidazoles
Microtrak, 96, 116
Midwives, 122, 198–99
Mineral deficiencies, 214–15
Misdiagnosis, 184
Molds, 22, 24, 108
Monilia/Moniliasis, 7, 8
  see also Vaginal yeast
    infections
  see also Candida albicans
Moniliasis, 7, 8
Monistat, 82, 119, 165, 173,
    175, 204, 206, 239, 250,
    251–52
Monistat Derm, 206
Mood swings, 106, 224
Mouthwash, antifungal, 59–60
Mucous membranes, 7–8, 31,
    32, 46, 51
Mucus (vaginal)
  tracking, 89–90
Multiple infections, 71, 90–91,
    110, 195

Mushrooms, 27, 30
  see also Molds
  see also Fungus
Mycolog II (cream), 204
Mycology, 9, 33–34
Mycosis, 7, 8
Mycostatin, 178
Mycostatin Oral Suspension,
  207

Nails, infections of, 5, 33, 178,
  182
Nipples, 33, 68, 73
  infected, 191, 206
Nizoral, 182
Nondrug antifungals, 149, 150,
  183–91
Nonspecific vaginitis, 102–3,
  188
Nursing mothers, 46, 181
  see also Breast-feeding
Nutrition, 67, 103, 203
  guidelines for, 215–21
  poor, as disposing condition,
    40, 48–49, 64–66, 106,
    136, 212
  in pregnancy, 197
Nystatin, 59–60, 69, 82, 107,
    108, 172, 174, 175–79,
    181, 195, 204
  oral, 145, 146–47, 207
  use during pregnancy, 199
  in prevention, 239
Nystex, 146
Nystex Oral Suspension, 207

Odors (vaginal), 87
  see also Discharge, odor
Opportunistic infections, 34,
    38, 39, 48
Oral contraceptives, 6, 15, 89,
    189
  and chronic yeast infections,
    71–73

as predisposing condition,
    11–12, 34, 39, 44–47,
    106, 121, 136
  stopping use of, 225–26
Oral sex, 53, 58–60, 93, 98, 99
Oral thrush, 8, 10, 33, 36–37,
    105
  abrasions/irritations and, 60–
    61
  gentian violet in treatment of,
    190
  in infants, 67–68, 73, 201,
    205–8
  in men, 5
  transmission of, 59
  treatment of, 178
Orithrush, 59
  mouthwash, 206
  Vaginal Douch Concentrate,
    188
Ortho (co.), 155, 239
Ortho Personal Lubricant, 228
Ortho Pharmaceuticals (co.),
    155, 175, 239, 250
Over-the-counter drugs, 172,
    173–75
  reclassification to, 249–53

Pap smear, 101, 102, 112, 113–
    16
  frequency of, 123
Pasteur, Louis, 28–29
Pasteurization, 28–29, 30
Pathogens, 34, 92, 110, 200
  yeast as, 32, 33, 36
Pelvic exam, 83, 112, 113, 116,
    122, 123
Pelvic inflammatory disease
    (PID), 96, 169
Pelvis, female, 114f
  male, 194f
Penicillin, 24, 29–30, 96, 238
  ingested with food, 43
Penis, 192, 230
  candidiasis of, 54, 57

pH (vagina), 51, 52, 72, 89, 102, 138, 153, 154, 226–27, 231, 239
  alkaline, 48, 49
  of aloe, 167
  altered, 45–46, 215
  fluctuations in, 76
  tests for, 209
  in vaginitis, 95, 96
Pharmaceutical companies, 14, 15, 121, 144, 150
Physiological change, 34, 36, 92, 112, 191
  as predisposing factor, 135–36
Pill (the), *see* Oral contraceptives
Plant life, 21, 22–23
Polyene antibiotics, 172, 174*t*
Polysystemic Chronic Candidiasis (PSCC), 105–8
Postmenopausal women, 2, 81
Povidine-iodine, 100, 184, 188–90, 199
Predisposing conditions, 6, 12, 15, 16, 17, 32, 34, 35–69, 82, 118, 134, 136–37
  elimination of, 151
Pregnancy, 10, 88, 89, 92, 112, 209, 216
  avoiding drugs in, 94, 96
  douching during, 170
  gonorrhea and, 98
  herpes and, 100
  homeopathic treatment in, 163
  as predisposing condition, 39, 45, 49–52, 106, 136, 196–200, 212
  susceptibility in, 37
  treatment during, 149, 151, 159, 179, 181, 187, 189–90, 196–200
  and yeast infections, 6, 12, 50, 68, 72
Premenstrual period, 6

Premenstrual symptoms, 75–76
Premenstrual syndrome (PMS), 49, 76, 79, 89, 106, 224
Prescription drugs, 38–39, 92, 96, 104, 112, 123, 211–12
  research studies on, 150
  in treatment of oral thrush, 207
  use during pregnancy, 199
Prevention, 16, 63, 151, 187–88, 211–40
  of diaper rash, 201–2
  douching in, 170
  lactobacilli in, 210
  in oral sex, 59–60
  of oral thrush, 206
  during pregnancy, 198
  for sexual partner, 191–96
Prevention tips, 213–14, 224, 233
Primary cure rate, *see* Cure rates
Primary resistance, 179
Progesterone, 45, 47, 50, 197, 209
Prophylactic therapy, 81–82, 120, 145, 210
Psychosomatic illness, 79, 124
Pulsatilla (windflower), 164, 165

Rash(es), 90, 193
  see also Diaper rash
Recurrence, 4, 13–14, 15, 73, 78, 120, 124, 125, 137, 252
  of herpes, 99–100
  during pregnancy, 196
  sexual transmission and, 196
  solving problem of, 133
  and treatment of sexual partner, 58
Recurrence rates, 3, 13, 14, 57, 121, 144, 150
  with imidazoles, 181–82

Resistance, 12, 34, 78, 89, 209–10
Ringworm, 105, 159, 182

Sanitary napkins, 48, 77, 102, 231
Schering-Plough (co.), 250–51, 253
Selenium, 64, 214–15
Self-diagnosis, 15, 16, 90, 91, 165, 251, 252–53
   mistakes in, 184
Self-help books, 3, 4, 122
Self-treatment, 3, 4, 149–71
   during pregnancy, 199
Semen, 6, 48, 89
Seminal fluid, 56, 227
Sexual activity, 6–7, 87, 112, 134, 226, 227–28
   and nonspecific vaginitis, 103
   and pH, 227
   see also Intercourse
Sexual arousal, 6, 48, 88, 227
Sexual partner(s), 124, 173, 180
   hygiene, 230
   new, multiple, 92, 103, 112
   treatment/prevention for, 53, 54, 56, 57, 58, 74–75, 94, 95, 96, 97, 98, 104, 149, 191–96
Sexual transmission, 39, 52–58, 73–75, 136, 191–92
   gardnerella vaginitis, 95
   oral, anal, lesbian sex, 58–60
   trichomonas, 93
   vaginitis, 89, 103–4
   yeast infections, 1, 12, 193
Sexually transmitted diseases, 11, 97–98
   screening for, 195–96
Side effects
   antibiotics, 237–38, 239
   boric acid, 160–61
   caprylic acid, 186–87
   imidazoles, 179–80

immunosuppressants, 63
ketoconazole, 183
metronidazole, 94
nystatin, 178
oral antifungals, 147
oral contraceptives, 73
povidone-iodine, 189
in treatment of oral thrush, 207
Skin infections, 32, 33, 34, 178, 190
Skin irritations, 71, 106, 203, 227–28
   see also Abrasional irritations
Sorbic acid, 184, 188
Spermicides, 61, 90, 225, 231
Spontaneous generation, 28
Sprouting mycelial form (yeast), 84, 85–86
Squibb (co.), 204, 207
Sterility, 96, 97
Steroids, 12, 33, 62–63
Stress, 12, 76, 89, 94, 103, 134, 213
   and diet, 221
   herpes and, 99
   menstrual, 48, 49
   as predisposing condition, 40, 64–66, 212
   and sugar cravings, 216
   as warning, 223–24
Sugar(s), 64–65, 76, 80, 197, 198, 202, 208, 212
   reducing intake of, 215–17
Sugar cravings, 216–17
Summer's Eve, 189
Suppositories, 2, 82
   antifungal, 172, 195
   boric acid, 160, 161
   gentian violet, 190
   homeopathic, 164, 165
   imidazoles, 180, 181
   lactobacilli, 210
   povidone-iodine, 189
   use during pregnancy, 199

Susceptibility (yeast), 2, 32–33,
      64, 73, 76, 78, 209, 212
   during menstruation, 231–32
   during pregnancy, 196, 197
   reduction of, 209
Symptom relief, 15, 39, 84, 118,
      120, 133, 144, 212
   with antifungals, 173
   home remedies in, 152, 153,
      168t
   multiple courses of therapy
      for, 196
Symptoms, 1, 38, 39, 71, 86, 87,
      88–89, 90, 92, 193
   atrophic vaginitis, 52, 101
   chlamydia, 96
   doderlein cytolysis, 102
   gardnerella vaginitis, 95
   general, 111, 112
   gonorrhea, 97
   herpes, 98, 99
   in men, 56, 57
   before and during menstrua-
      tion, 47–48, 75–76
   nonspecific vaginitis, 103
   oral thrush, 67
   persisting, 182
   suppression of, 163
   trichomonas vaginitis, 93
Syphilis, 33, 92, 126

Tampons, 48, 61, 77, 89, 102,
      227, 230–32
   gentian violet, 190–91
   O.B. brand, 141–42, 155, 171
   super-absorbent, 77, 89
Terazol, 175
Terconazole, 172, 174, 179, 181
Tests, testing, 112–17
   false negatives, 97
Tetracyclines, 41, 97, 137
Thiamine, 27, 214
Thrush, 7, 8, 9, 10, 37
   diaper, *see* Diaper rash

   gentian violet in treatment of,
      190
   transmission of, 53–54
   see also Oral thrush; Vaginal
      thrush
Tinactin, 204, 206
Tinea corporis, 182
Tobacco, 213, 219–20
Toxic Shock Syndrome (TSS),
      77, 171
Toxicity, 178, 179, 186
Transudation, 88
Treatment, 15, 16, 57, 104, 110,
      124, 128, 133–210
   atrophic vaginitis, 101
   doderlein cytolysis, 102
   failure of, 120
   future, 208–10
   herpes, 100
   ineffective, 16–17, 92, 112
   intravaginal, 141–42, 153–71
   nonmedical, 141
   nonspecific vaginitis, 103
   oral thrush, 206–07
   oral/topical, 145–46
   Polysystemic Chronic Candi-
      diasis, 107–08
   for special cases, 196–208
   of vagina, 120
   of yeast infections, 148t, 149
   see also Self-treatment; Sex-
      ual partner(s), treatment/
      prevention for
Treatment regimen(s), 145, 180,
      181, 185, 189
   see also Antibiotic therapy
Trichomonas, 89, 90, 91–94,
      116, 154, 188, 209, 225,
      226
Triggers, *see* Predisposing
      conditions

Underlying conditions, 3, 78,
      82, 101–8

Underwear, 229–30, 232, 233
Urinary tract infection, 93
Urination
  frequent, 51
  painful, 14, 90, 92, 93, 99, 201

Vagina, 5, 31, 88, 143
  clean, ventilated, 232, 233
  healthy, 86, 225
  self-cleansing, 37, 38, 169,
    226
  treatment of, 120
Vaginal area (diagram), 115*f*
Vaginal candidiasis/candidosis,
    see Vaginal yeast
    infections
Vaginal environment, 46, 72,
    78, 151, 226
  care of, 226
  changes in, 6, 197
  effect of semen on, 227
  healthy, 86, 87
Vaginal moniliasis
  see Vaginal yeast infections
Vaginal sprays, 89
Vaginal thrush, 8, 10, 37–38, 50,
    54
Vaginal yeast infections, 1–8,
    15, 32–33, 70–71, 90, 91,
    105
  chronic, 79, 80, 123, 191–92
  cycle of, 3–4, 12–14
  defined, 1
  diagnosis of, 82–86
  as diagnostic tool, 105
  emotional cost of, 123–30
  four-step program for, 5,
    134–49
  history of, 8–11
  incidence of, 11–12, 50
  as indicators of other prob-
    lems, 104–08
  in infancy, 66–69
  myths of, 16, 71–82

  as normal part of being fe-
    male, 79–80
  physical and emotional as-
    pects of, 109–30
  Pill (the) and, 71–73
  substances used for treating,
    148*t*, 149
  terminology of, 7–8
  untreated, 78–79
  women's monopoly on, 5–7
  see also Predisposing condi-
    tions; Recurrence;
    Symptoms
Vaginitis, 7, 8, 49–50, 70–108,
    111, 112
  cause of, 10, 31
  guidelines for avoiding, 103–
    04
  Pill-associated, 225
  recurrent, 54, 56, 106
  term, 87
  yeast/non-yeast, 87–103
Vaseline, 228
Venereal disease, 53
  see also Sexually transmitted
    diseases
Vinegar, 150, 152, 153–56, 157,
    231
Viral infections, 36, 98
Virgins, 7, 93
Viruses, 29, 238
Vitamin/mineral supplement,
    220–21
Vitamins, 27, 64, 65, 140, 141,
    213, 214
Vulvovaginal dandidiasis
  see Vaginal yeast infections

Wet mount, *see* Pap smear

Yeast(s), 10, 16, 24–28, 32, 38,
    39, 50, 76, 225
  as cause of infections, 82–86

Yeast(s) (*cont.*)
  as commensal, 36
  food value of, 27–28
  gastrointestinal, 31, 144–51
  and infants, 200–01, 202–03
  pathological, 83–86
  reducing vaginal, 143
Yeast/bacteria ratio, 69
  disturbance in, 137–39, 142
Yeast cell(s), 24
Yeast "die-off," *see* Herxhei-
    mer reaction
Yeast eradication
  four-point program for, 5,
    134–49
Yeast form
  as diagnostic tool, 84–85
Yeast-Free Diet, 44, 234–36
Yeast-Gard, 164–65

Yeast growth, 5, 33, 41, 48
Yeast infections, *see* Vaginal
    yeast infections
Yeast load, 85–86
Yeast organisms, 192–93
  transmission of, 73
  warm, moist environment
    for, 5, 33, 49, 61, 67, 77,
    206
Yeast vaginitis, *see* Vaginal
    yeast infections
Yeast-X, 165
Yogurt, 139, 150, 152, 156–57,
    199, 239
  in douches, 155
  intravaginal, 141–42

Zinc, 64, 65, 100